Learning to use
THE PROCESS OF
NURSING

NANCY ROPER is the author of *Principles of Nursing, Man's Anatomy, Physiology, Health and Environment* and the *Churchill Livingstone Nurses Dictionary*. She trained at the General Infirmary in Leeds and later spent 15 years at the Cumberland Infirmary School of Nursing as Principal Tutor. In 1970, following a period of full-time writing, she was awarded a research fellowship from the Commonwealth Nurses' War Memorial Fund. The research, into clinical experience in nurse education, was undertaken from the Nursing Research Unit at the University of Edinburgh and gained the M.Phil degree. From 1975 to 1978 she was Nursing Officer (Research) at the Scottish Home and Health Department.

WIN LOGAN is Head of Department of Health and Nursing Studies, Glasgow College of Technology, Scotland. She was Executive Director of the International Council of Nurses (ICN) from 1978–80. She had already gained considerable knowledge and experience of nursing internationally, having worked or served as a consultant in Canada, the USA, Malaysia and Iraq. In 1971–2 she acted as Chief Nursing Officer at the newly created Ministry of Health in Abu Dhabi. Prior to moving to the ICN she worked for 4 years at the Scottish Home and Health Department where she had responsibility for nursing education. She took to that post experience gained from a 12-year term of office, first as lecturer and latterly as senior lecturer, in the Department of Nursing Studies at the University of Edinburgh. She is an arts graduate of that university and did her basic nurse education at the Royal Infirmary of Edinburgh.

ALISON TIERNEY is a graduate nurse and was one of the first nurses in the UK to gain a doctoral degree. Her PhD was obtained for research done in the field of mental handicap nursing while holding a Nursing Research Fellowship awarded by the Scottish Home and Health Department. From 1973–80 she was a lecturer in the Department of Nursing Studies at the University of Edinburgh. Amongst other things, her post involved her in the development of the foundation nursing course for first-year students and in the clinical supervision of students at various stages in the degree/nursing programme. During 1976 and 1977 she acted as nurse adviser to the Edinburgh Medical Group research project, set up to develop methods of studying medical ethics and moral issues in health care.

Nancy Roper, Win Logan and Alison Tierney are the joint authors of *The Elements of Nursing*.

Learning to use
THE PROCESS OF
NURSING

NANCY ROPER
M.Phil RGN RSCN RNT

WINIFRED W. LOGAN
MA DNS (Educ.) RGN RNT

ALISON J. TIERNEY
B.Sc (Soc.Sc.-Nurs.) PhD RGN

CHURCHILL LIVINGSTONE
EDINBURGH LONDON MELBOURNE AND NEW YORK 1981

CHURCHILL LIVINGSTONE
Medical Division of Longman Group Limited

Distributed in the United States of America by Churchill Livingstone
Inc., 19 West 44th Street, New York, N.Y. 10036, and by associated
companies, branches and representatives throughout the world.

First published 1981

ISBN 0 443 02234 8

British Library Cataloguing in Publication Data
Roper, Nancy
    Learning to use the process of nursing.
  1. Health
  2. Nursing
  I. Title   II. Logan, Winifred W
  III. Tierney, Alison J
  613′.02′4613   RT67   80–41460

Printed in Singapore by Kyodo Shing Loong Printing Industries Pte Ltd

Preface

In our previous book *The Elements of Nursing* we presented a model for nursing which, developed from a model of living, has as its focus activities of living (ALs). This model provides a way for nurses to consider patients' problems related to their everyday living activities. Therefore, nursing is viewed as helping patients to solve, alleviate, cope with, or prevent problems with activities of living, rather than as treating patients with specific disease conditions, the approach implicit in a 'medical model'.

The concept of the process of nursing—involving the phases commonly called assessment, planning, implementation and evaluation—is incorporated within our model for nursing. Our main hope for *The Elements of Nursing* is that it will help nurses and nurse learners to develop a way of thinking about nursing as an activity which has as its focus patients' problems with ALs, and which involves for each patient, a problem-solving approach.

This book is a logical extension. It attempts to help nurses to see how this way of thinking about nursing can be applied to practice. We hope this small book will be useful to nurses, nurse learners and nurse teachers—indeed anyone who is interested in learning to use the process of nursing.

After an introduction which outlines the model for nursing and the process of nursing, there follows a series of presentations. Each aims to exemplify a particular aspect of application: for example, one looks at identifying patients' problems, another at planning in the context of patient teaching. However it is not a theoretical approach but a practical one. For this reason, each example has as its focus a particular patient. We have selected patients from all stages of the life-span and with different kinds of health problems affecting the ALs in various ways. The patients presented are not 'real' but are realistic and represent the kinds of patients that nurse learners encounter in even their early clinical experience.

In preparing this book we have come to realise that the process of nursing, far from being a simple activity, is in fact a highly complex one. The experienced nurse, able to use the process competently and confidently, needs to remember that it is an approach to nursing which does need to be *learned*. However, there can be no doubt that use of the process in the short-term provides the means of individualising nursing and, in the long-term, analysis of the accumulated data base would further our understanding of nursing.

Edinburgh, 1981 NR, WL, AT

Contents

1

Introduction

A MODEL FOR NURSING

In order to write *The Elements of Nursing* a particular mode of thinking about nursing had to be agreed upon, and it was decided to use as a starting point the model for nursing developed previously by one of the authors (Roper, 1976). This model for nursing is based on a model of living which focuses on *Activities of Living* (ALs). Twelve ALs were included in the model:

- maintaining a safe environment
- communicating
- breathing
- eating and drinking
- eliminating
- personal cleansing and dressing
- controlling body temperature
- mobilising
- working and playing
- expressing sexuality
- sleeping
- dying

To use ALs as the focus of a nursing model is based on the idea that people who are in need of nursing have some sort of health problem, actual or potential, which has an effect on everyday living—on the carrying out of *activities of living*.

It is this same model for nursing which has been used as the framework for the development of this book and, because the model incorporates the process of nursing, a discussion of the process follows.

THE PROCESS OF NURSING

The process—usually described as having four phases: assessment, planning, implementation and evaluation—is not new in nursing; the 'good nurse' has always used it. Often, however, she did not analyse what she was doing,

nor did she verbalise the phases of the process as she carried out each nursing activity, so some learners found it difficult to appreciate the rapidly executed cognitive aspects of the task observed. Learners were often unaware that the experienced nurse had selected out of several possible alternatives, one particular regime for a particular patient, and were therefore unable to comprehend the reason.

Nor was the rationale apparent to the non-nurses who studied the work of nurses in the 1950s and '60s. To them, much of nurses' work appeared simply as 'tasks' such as filling in patients' admission forms; preparing for, serving and clearing away after meals; and doing domestic work in the wards. In the reports of these studies the term 'non-nursing' tasks was introduced and it was recommended, for example, that ward clerks and domestic supervisors should be appointed and that an independent meal-serving system should be introduced. The wisdom of such developments is now being questioned in the light of current reconsideration of nursing.

Also nurses did not commit to paper their rapid thinking about assessing, planning, implementing and evaluating. If all nurses begin to document and retain nursing data, it will not only be useful for nursing subsequent patients, but it will provide evidence of:
- nursing's body of knowledge
- the value and prestige of the nurse-initiated components of nursing
- the evaluated effectiveness of specific nursing interventions
- the decision-making aspects underlying nursing activities, a criterion used by managers when assessing status and earnings

ASSESSMENT

Activities of living (ALs) can be used as the criteria for which assessment data is collected. Data about the patient's

ALs need not be collected in any particular order and in some circumstances not all ALs need to be considered. It is often inadvisable to collect very detailed information at the first encounter with a patient; indeed it is likely that further pertinent information will be forthcoming at each interaction with the patient as increasing rapport is established. Of course, in life-threatening emergency situations, only minimal essential data is collected before the patient is transferred to the operating theatre or before life-saving measures are implemented.

Whatever type of admission form, assessment form, nursing history or nursing Kardex is used for recording purposes, the nurse needs to be very sensitive about where, when and how she collects information from patients. Part of the skill of nursing is recognising when, and knowing how to collect information.

Some patients may not want to divulge information about certain aspects of their daily living, wishing to retain as much privacy as possible. The nurse can explain that certain information is essential if the necessary treatment is to be provided and that other information may be relevant in identifying potential, as well as actual, health problems. Nurses who have used nursing assessments usually experience favourable patients' reactions to the opportunity of giving information and talking with a nurse.

However, it may also be important to reassure patients that information given to nurses is regarded as confidential. Confidentiality is often a loosely used word these days; rather than using this term, it may be advisable to state exactly where information will be stored and who has access to it, reassuring the patient that information is confined to the health care team.

Some hospitals are experimenting with patient-completed assessment forms. Aspinall (1975) carried out a comparative study and found that the data thus obtained compared favourably with information collected from the nursing interview. But obviously not all patients would be able or willing to participate in such an exercise.

To help readers to develop skills in assessing, a broad view will be given of the sort of information relevant to consider in a nursing assessment. Examples are given of the type of questions that the nurse in her role of assessor might bear in mind when interacting with a patient. The patient need not be asked all the questions; in fact the nurse will obtain many 'answers' by astute observation—some of which of course will need to be confirmed by the patient. The list of questions is not exhaustive and many others will be seen to be appropriate as the nurse becomes more skilled at assessing patients. The objectives in collecting data about patients' ALs are to discover:
- previous routines
- what the patient can do for himself
- what the patient cannot do for himself
- problems (actual/potential) and previous coping mechanisms

Assessing ability to maintain a safe environment is of particular importance if the patient has any sensory impairment: poor vision, poor hearing, inability to smell, or loss of peripheral sensation. How does the blind person prevent injury? What precautions does the deaf person take to avoid accident? Has the patient who cannot smell developed any compensatory activities, or taken any precautions, to make his environment safe? What activities does the paraplegic patient carry out to prevent pressure sores? Whether they are in hospital or at home, what can physically and/or mentally handicapped patients do to keep their environment safe? Assessing ability to maintain a safe environment is an important function of the community nurses, especially those visiting children or elderly people. Is the floor trip-free? Are the hygiene standards sufficient to prevent infection? Are fires guarded? Are medicines, poisons and sharp instruments stored safely?

Assessing communicating skills can take place at every interaction between nurse and patient. It has to be remembered that communicating is one of the ALs which is very much affected by such factors as stage of development, level of intelligence, personality traits and current mood. The following examples are general questions which will apply to most adults. Can he see and hear adequately? If not, is there dysfunction of right or left eye/ear or both? What factors does he find helpful/unhelpful when people are talking with him? Does he use any corrective aids? Are they in good working order? Is his speech audible, coherent, fluent, confident, inaudible, incoherent, interrupted in its flow, nervous? Does he appear to have a limited/average/extensive vocabulary? Can he read and write? Does he appear to be comfortable/uncomfortable with eye contact? Does he gesticulate excessively/acceptably/sparingly? Is he gregarious by nature or more fond of his own company?

Assessing a patient's breathing may involve simply ensuring that breathing has not stopped or, more usually for various reasons, counting and recording the number of respirations per minute. Given that the patient is breathing, the nurse needs to discover: Does he have any difficulty with breathing? Does he have any pain or discomforts associated with breathing? Can he describe the pain? When does it occur? What increases/decreases the pain? For other patients the nurse will need to ask: Does he cough? If so, when? Does coughing produce sputum? Can he describe the sputum? What increases/decreases the coughing? Does the atmosphere at work exacerbate the coughing? Is his breathing ever 'wheezy'? Does he get colds often/sometimes/seldom/never? Does he smoke? If so, does he smoke cigarettes, cigars, a pipe? How many cigarettes, cigars, or how much tobacco? Does he smoke daily? What factors increase/decrease his usual smoking habits? At what age did he start smoking? Has he ever given it up? If so, for how long? What made him start again? What does he know about the ill effects of smoking?

Assessing eating and drinking routines is a necessary part of an admission assessment so that related nursing can be planned appropriately. What is the person's usual diet, dietary likes and dislikes? Are any dietary modifications observed? If so, are these medical, religious, sociocultural or personal-choice modifications? Is he able to eat and drink independently? Are any aids needed to maintain independence? If the patient is a child, exact details of his dependence/independence will be necessary. Does the patient have any problems or discomforts associated with eating and drinking? If so, can he describe them, their relationship to food/fluid intake, and what relieves them? Is he overnourished/well nourished/undernourished? Is his weight in keeping with his height, build and age? What are his usual eating and drinking routines: does he eat alone or with others; where does he usually eat and drink? Because most people enjoy talking about this AL, information about it is usually relatively easy to obtain.

Assessing a patient's eliminating habits is a necessary nursing function even though his current health problem is not associated with bowel or urinary dysfunction. But there may well be a long-term problem with constipation or recurrent cystitis and this may be elicited from the assessment. Many people find it embarrassing to talk about elimination and the nurse needs to broach the topic with sensitivity and phrase the questions carefully to avoid embarrassment. The nurse can help the patient by saying that different people use different words (water, urine, voiding; stool, faeces, bowel movement, bowels open) and using the ones with which the patient is familiar. At what time does he pass urine? What factors increase/decrease this frequency? Can he estimate how much he passes each time? What factors increase/decrease this amount? Does he have any difficulty in passing urine? Can he describe it? What increases/decreases the difficulty? Can he describe the urine? What is his normal bowel habit? What factors increase/decrease this frequency? Can he describe the faeces? Does he have any problems or discomforts associated with defaecation? From patients who excrete via a stoma, the nurse will discover how they cope at home, and whether or not they will continue to cope independently in hospital.

Assessing personal cleansing and dressing is possible by observing the results of these activities; ill-cared for clothes may be an indication of financial hardship or a lack of self-esteem which can characterise exhaustion or mental illness. Shabby but clean clothes may be an indication of financial hardship. Clothes inappropriate for the climatic conditions may be indicative of inability to appreciate or respond appropriately to changes in the temperature of the external environment. It may be tactful to preface questions about personal hygiene by a remark such as 'What do we need to know so that we interfere as little as possible with your usual hygiene habits?' As with all the ALs, the nurse needs to be sensitive and skilful at recognising a patient's discomfort; some people are embarrassed at revealing that their home does not have a bathroom, while others are proud to proclaim that all the family have kept themselves clean without a bathroom. The objective in nurses collecting information about patients' personal cleansing activities is to permit such usual routines as bathing, handwashing, hairwashing and mouth cleaning to continue—unless a routine is found to be prejudicial to health. In this instance, instruction may be necessary so the nursing plan should include appropriate aspects of health education.

Assessing control of body temperature is not as amenable to questioning as many of the other ALs, but data can be obtained by observation and measurement. Observation may reveal flushing of the skin, excessive perspiration, the presence of goose flesh, shivering, and excessively hot or cold hands and/or feet. If an accurate assessment of body temperature is required, this may be measured with a clinical thermometer.

When assessing mobilising, initially it is necessary to observe whether or not there are any apparent musculoskeletal abnormalities. But people vary enormously in their exercise habits related to home, work and play activities so it is important to broach these various aspects of mobilising with the patient. Lack of exercise can contribute to some kinds of health problems and again inclusion of remedial health education in the nursing plan may be relevant. The patient who has an obvious mobilising problem may have a walking aid or wheelchair, and this will make it easier to discuss how he copes and what help he needs. Questions can be asked about impaired movement and pain. For example, is there any stiffness of the joints? If so, which ones? Does he know what causes it? Does he have any muscular pain or discomfort? If so, where? What increases/decreases it? Does he have any joint pains? If so, which joints? What increases/decreases the pain?

Assessing working and playing routines is necessary because they may well have implications for nursing. What is the patient's occupation? Where does he work? Can he describe the working conditions? By the way he responds the nurse may well discover whether he finds work challenging or boring and she would recognise whether or not the working conditions might have contributed to his accident or illness. There may be cues indicating difficulty in work or social relationships because of personality problems and these may have contributed to the illness. How far from home is his work and by which means does he travel? How many hours does he work? Does he work overtime and if so, how much? How much time does he devote to playing activities? What are his hobbies? When did he last have a holiday from work? How does he feel about being absent from work? Will he be bored while off sick? Obtaining details of play activities is essential if the patient is a child: what stage of development has he reached? What are his favourite toys and books?

Assessment of the AL of expressing sexuality will require a different approach, according to circumstances. In a gynaecological or genito-urinary unit, it may be important for the nurse to obtain information about sexual function, and the effects of the patient's health problem on his/her sexual feelings. It is likely that a female patient admitted to hospital for treatment of a gynaecological complaint will expect to be asked, and be prepared to answer, fairly direct questions about her menstrual cycle, contraceptive practice, parity and pregnancies. In contrast, such questions understandably, might alarm and embarrass a patient admitted for treatment of varicose veins, for example! However, now that it is beginning to be understood that many different sorts of health problems may affect sexual function or feelings of sexuality, it is essential for nurses to be able to obtain relevant data which will help them to identify patients' problems and anxieties concerning this AL, if it is appropriate to do so.

Assessing sleeping routines at an early stage is important so that nurses have information on which to base nursing activities aimed at promoting sleep. Patients are not usually admitted to hospital because of a sleep problem as such, but adequate sleep is important for progress towards recovery, whatever the reason for admission. What is the patient's pre-sleep routine? At what time does he retire to bed? At what time does he usually go to sleep? Does he waken during the sleep period; if so, at what time does he waken? What does he do to get to sleep again? Does he consider himself a good/average/poor sleeper? Does he feel refreshed/unrefreshed on waking? What is his usual 'morning mood'? Does he have to adjust his sleep to shift work? Does he take sleeping pills: always/sometimes/seldom/never? If so, does he know which ones? Does he have them with him? What factors increase/decrease his sleep?

Assessing the needs of the dying and the dying person's relatives is a very important role of the nurse in hospital and in the community. Constant sensitivity and astute observation are necessary to recognise whether or not the patient/relative wants to talk about the many anxieties associated with death, dying and bereavement. Assessment of the specific nursing needs of the dying patient may be carried out in relation to each AL separately, as previously discussed.

Assessment, then, is not a once-only activity, or a rigid routine carried out at a particular time. It is a continuous or ongoing activity as nurses are constantly observing and interacting with patients. The main purpose of a nursing assessment is identification of the patients' actual or potential problems that are amenable to nursing help. Apart from the problems obvious to the patient, there can be a nurse-perceived problem of which the patient is unaware: for example, infestation with head lice. It must be noted so that it can be treated otherwise lice may be transmitted to others. In other instances, the patient may wish to decide whether or not the problem, not apparent to him, should be treated.

The data from assessment are analysed and the patients' problems, both actual and potential should be clearly stated. For each actual/potential problem a goal or patient outcome is then decided. Discussion with the patient whenever it is possible, and perhaps with his family, may help in stating feasible patient outcomes that can be anticipated. Patient outcomes are the goals or objectives of nursing intervention. They should be stated in observable and/or measurable terms so that they can be used as criteria in the 'evaluation phase' of nursing.

To give some examples, if a patient's problem is constipation, the patient outcome would be a return to the usual bowel habit in which stools are not difficult or painful to pass. If the problem is incontinence of urine the desirable patient outcome would be continence of urine. A potential problem for any patient whose mobility is severely restricted, whether he is in bed or in a chair, is the development of a deep vein thrombosis in the lower limb, the presence of which causes pain and inflammation. The patient outcome stated in observable terms would be unswollen, pain-free lower limbs at the same temperature as the rest of the skin.

PLANNING

A clear statement of the expected outcomes leads naturally into the second phase of the process, planning for nursing intervention to achieve the expected patient outcomes. Planning includes consideration of:

- available resources, such as:
  physical environment
  equipment
  personnel
- possible alternative nursing interventions

When planning for the most appropriate *physical environment*, a decision may have to be made as to whether the person would be best nursed at home or in hospital. Should the patient have an infection and have to be barrier nursed, a single room would be preferable to a shared one. Planning also includes details of such factors as the distance between the bed and the toilet if the patient has to make frequent visits.

Availability of suitable *equipment* can have an important effect on planning nursing. Variable height beds may help to prevent accident to frail and disabled patients. Aids to mobilising, such as walking frames and wheelchairs, may be necessary. Special utensils have to be considered when patients have certain physical problems with feeding.

Consideration of *available personnel* will include not only numbers of nursing staff but also their level of preparation and their previous nursing experience. This has to be related to the planned nursing activities and especially to the nursing workload. In the inevitable instances of shortage of nursing staff on a particular work shift, existing personnel must decide which nursing activities can safely be omitted for that shift. It is safer to do essential nursing activities well than to attempt all desirable activities and risk not only sub-standard nursing but a lowering of the nurses' morale due to lack of job satisfaction. When patients are nursed at home, or their transfer home from hospital is imminent, the availability of family and neighbours should be considered as a resource.

When patients are nursed at home information about available support services is needed. Such resources as home-helps, volunteer workers, night nursing staff, laundry services and meals-on-wheels may have to be considered.

Possible alternative nursing interventions may be determined by the availability of resources. Decisions have to be made about such things as, for example, should the patient use a commode at the bedside independently or walk 15 steps to the toilet assisted by two nurses? Walking would perhaps best meet the patient's mobility needs but it involves two nurses at the required times. Choice of intervention may also be made on the basis of evidence of best known effectiveness: for example, regular relief of pressure is known to be preferable to an alternative commonly in use—'pressure care rounds'.

Having considered the resources, the next procedure is to make decisions about what the nurse and (when possible) the patient agree to do to achieve the expected outcomes related to each of the patient's problems. For those activities which the patient agrees to do, the associated nursing activity is supervision. *A nursing plan* is then made of all the necessary nursing activities stated in sufficient detail so that any other nurse, on reading the plan, would be aware of and carry out the planned nursing activities. There is no argument against this being essential since no one nurse can be on duty throughout the 24 hours and sufficient detail of the plans made for each patient cannot possibly be conveyed in verbal reports.

A nursing plan is not a static thing but requires continual revision as additional data are collected from ongoing assessment. Also, when evaluation reveals that an expected outcome has not been achieved for a particular patient's problem, there may well have to be a change in the nursing activities and this must be recorded in the nursing plan.

Social changes which have affected the nursing profession, such as decreased working hours, and an increase in both annual leave and the use of part-time staff, have made it essential for nurses to develop the skill of communicating by writing adequate nursing plans. If such trends continue, it may well be that the nursing plan will assume even greater importance as a means of communication between nurses. And furthermore, assessing a patient and writing a nursing plan help the nurse and patient to know each other. This, in turn, aids the establishment of a satisfactory nurse/patient relationship, the unique basis of the nursing contribution to a patient's health care.

IMPLEMENTATION

The third phase of the process of nursing is actually carrying out the prepared plan. A day-to-day record must be made of the nursing activities implemented: when they were carried out, and by whom, together with any relevant information (e.g., the patient may have experienced nausea soon after administration of the analgesic drug prescribed for him). An 'implementation sheet', 'flow chart' or 'record sheet' can be used for the purpose of recording the nursing activities implemented. Whatever the format, it is important for nurses to consider this recording as a data-collecting exercise. The data must be retained as they will become nursing's data bank on which retrospective research can be carried out to fill many of the gaps in our knowledge of nursing.

EVALUATION

It is difficult to justify the existence of nursing if it cannot be demonstrated that it benefits the recipient in specific ways, hence the fourth phase in the process of nursing, evaluation. The expected patient outcomes, already stated, are the criteria used in evaluation; without them, evaluation is a misnomer. Some nurses are confused about assessing and evaluating; some of the skills used are common to both activities, but evaluating involves comparison against an objective—the stated patient outcome. When the expected outcomes are not achieved, there has to be reassessment of that problem with the patient, and consequent recycling of the process of nursing as illustrated in Figure 1.1 on page 6.

At the Congress in Tokyo in 1977, the president of the International Council of Nurses chose the watchword *accountability* for nurses for the next quadrennium. The two crucial issues in nursing accountability are: statement of expected patient outcomes and evaluation of whether or

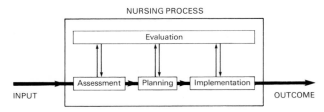

Fig 1.1 The process of nursing

not they have been achieved. They are crucial because the evaluative component of nursing cannot take place unless preceded by a statement of expectation. By using the process of nursing, nurses should be able to render accountability for the service which they provide.

REFERENCES

Aspinall M J 1975 Development of a patient-completed questionnaire and its comparison with the nursing interview. Nursing Research 24 (5): 377–381

Roper N 1976 Clinical experience in nurse education. Churchill Livingstone, Edinburgh

Roper N, Logan W, Tierney A 1980 The elements of nursing. Churchill Livingstone, Edinburgh

SUGGESTED READING

Brearley P 1978 Confidentiality—the need for a code of practice. Nursing Times 74 (12) March 23: 505

Clarke R 1979 Assessment in psychiatric hospitals. Nursing Times 75 (14) April 5: 590–592

Crow J 1979 The nursing process—a framework for care studies. Nursing Times 75 (32) August 9: 1362–1365

Kershaw J E M 1979 Standard care plans. Nursing Times 75 (33) August 16: 1413–1416

Kratz C R (ed) 1979 The nursing process. Bailliere Tindall, London

Luker K A 1979 A framework for the nursing process: problem-oriented recordings. Nursing Times 75 (35) August 30: 1488–1490

Mackie L et al 1979 Revitalising the nursing care plan. Nursing Times 75 (34) August 23: 1440–1450

Nursing Times Reprint 1978 Rediscovering the patient. Macmillan Journals, London

2

Patient assessment form

The Patient Assessment Form used throughout this book has as its rationale, recording of the patient's biographical and health data on the left-hand side and data about the patient's ALs on the right-hand side (Fig. 2.1, pp. 8–9). As will be shown in the 11 presentations, these two sets of data do have relevance to each other. Use of each side of the form will be discussed separately.

BIOGRAPHICAL AND HEALTH DATA

Because there may be two patients with the same *surname* it is necessary to write out the *forenames* in long hand and to avoid using initials for any of them. It is customary in some hospitals to ask the patient what form of address he would prefer the staff to use because being addressed in the usual way can help a patient to retain his sense of personal identity and dignity.

All cities have their affluent and disadvantaged areas so an *address* can alert the staff to possible problems which the patient might have on discharge, with ALs such as mobilising or maintaining a safe environment. An address may give an indication of status and income which could be relevant to the nursing plan, e.g., a patient in the low income group who requires an expensive high protein diet.

Likewise the *type of accommodation* could well have relevance to the nursing plan; if a chronically breathless patient lives in a fourth floor flat that does not have a lift, arrangement of an early appointment with the medical social worker will be a necessary nursing activity. When patients are on diuretic drugs the type of toilet accommodation is obviously relevant.

Information about *family/others* who live at the patient's address may reveal that he lives alone, a factor which could influence the planning of his rehabilitation and the date of his discharge. It could also inform the staff of his anxiety and fear about the house being unoccupied, or especially in the winter months about problems such as burst water

pipes. In other instances, should a telephone call have to be made by a nurse to this address, it is important for her to know to whom she might be speaking.

The name of the *next of kin*, is, of course, essential information; even the knowledge that there is no next of kin is important and relevant. As one of the presentations demonstrates, a patient separated from his wife did not want her to be contacted without his permission.

Information about the *significant others* in a patient's life can have relevance to planning the patient's nursing. The adolescent diabetic in the presentation 'Identifying patients' learning needs' (Ch. 5) reveals her lack of knowledge about diabetes and heredity, and pregnancy, while talking about her boyfriend. This important information enabled the teaching plan to include these subjects together with discussion of the availability of genetic counselling. In another of the presentations, collection of this section of biographical data reveals that the patient would not be having any visitors during his short hospital stay.

The patient's *occupation* may not only affect the planning of a rehabilitation programme for him but also alert the nurse to think about how for instance a low income might be affecting his family and she could offer to make an appointment with the medical social worker. On the other hand, the occupation could be a contributory factor to the reason for admission, e.g., dust from coal mining being a precursor to chronic respiratory disease.

It is important for nurses to know of any *religious beliefs and practices* which have implications for the nursing plan. The patient may or may not wish to attend the services in the hospital chapel, or participate in a ward communion service, or be visited by a particular hospital chaplain or his own minister of religion. Religious beliefs can have direct bearing on the ALs of eating, drinking, personal cleansing and dressing.

Collection of *health data* can be carried out prior to the assessment interview, indeed they and many of the biographical data can be collected from the patient's case

Patient Assessment Form

Date of admission   Date of assessment

Surname   Forenames

Male [ ]   Age [ ]   Single/Married/Widowed   Prefers to be addressed as

Female   Other

                             Date of birth

Address of usual residence

Type of accommodation

Family/Others at this residence

Next of kin   Name   Address

                     Relationship   Tel. no.

Significant others   Relatives/Dependents

                          Helpers

                          Visitors

Occupation

Religious beliefs and relevant practices

Patient's perception of current health status

Reason for admission/referral

Medical diagnosis

Past medical history

Allergies   Significant life crises

Fig. 2.1 A sample of a Patient Assessment Form (the year has been purposefully omitted from the date of admission)

Assessment of Activities of Living

Date

AL | Usual routines:
what he/she can and cannot do independently

Patient's problems
(actual/potential)
(p) = potential

- Maintaining
a safe
environment

- Communicating

- Breathing

- Eating and
drinking

- Eliminating

- Personal
cleansing and
dressing

- Controlling
body
temperature

- Mobilising

- Working
and playing

- Expressing
sexuality

- Sleeping

- Dying

notes which usually results in a more relaxed interview. Information about the patient's health data permits the nurse to gain understanding of his knowledge about, and his attitude to his health status. It is important for nurses to know his perception of his current health status: e.g., his understanding of the nature of a chronic disorder. It is useful for nurses to know his understanding of the reason for his admission, for instance whether or not he knows that he has been scheduled for an investigation under general anaesthetic and not an operation. He may or may not know his medical diagnosis and past medical history, and in any case these should be checked with the medical notes.

Allergies are an important consideration. There are so many things (adhesive bandages, particular foods, pollens, feathers and drugs) to which people are allergic and it is important to record these.

It is useful to know whether the patient has undergone recently any *significant life crisis* such as starting new employment, changing house or school, marriage, divorce or bereavement; it is known that such crises can affect health adversely.

The biographical and health data, collected as described, in addition to providing essential information about the patient, will suggest topics obviously requiring further exploration in the more detailed assessment of each AL.

ACTIVITIES OF LIVING DATA

On the right-hand side of the patient assessment form, data about each of the patient's ALs is recorded. In Chapter 1 there are examples of the sort of questions to bear in mind at the assessment interview and indeed at all times, since it cannot be too strongly stressed that assessment is an ongoing process. The objective is to discover the patient's previous routines, what he can and cannot do for himself in relation to each AL. After analysis of the data the patient's problems are identified and written on the right-hand side of the form. Potential problems are identified by the sign (p).

To give readers further help with collecting AL data, the summary charts from *The Elements of Nursing* are reproduced on pages 11 to 22. They were devised as an aide memoire at the end of discussion of each AL. In addition to listing factors relevant in assessment, they include patients' possible problems and the kind of nursing activities related to patients' problems with that AL.

Maintaining a safe environment

ASSESSMENT

Influencing factors
  stage of development
  physical factors
    hearing
    seeing
    touching
    tasting
    smelling
    dizziness
    mobilising ability
    mobility aids
  psychological factors
    intelligence
    knowledge of and attitudes to
      safety at home/work/play
      road safety
      smoking
      handwashing
      spread of infection
      medicines/poisons
      alcoholism
    personality and temperament
    awareness of danger
  socio-economic factors
    housing
    social class
    economic status

Standard of safety in the home
  tidiness
  flooring
  water supply
  heat and light supply
  toilet facilities
  storage of medicines/poisons
  state of stairs/steps/paths
  hygiene standards
  fire precautions

Evidence of safety when working and playing
  protective clothing
  smoking habits
  safety of equipment
  safe use of equipment
  safety of environment
  safe behaviour

ANALYSIS OF DATA

IDENTIFICATION OF PATIENTS' PROBLEMS

Change of environment
  unfamiliar environment
  noise
  nervousness
  exposure to micro-organisms
  exposure to hazards, such as oxygen
    therapy

Change of routine
  cleansing routines
  taking medications

Change of mode
  visual impairment/loss
  aural impairment/loss
  smelling and tasting
    impairment/loss
  mobilising impairment/loss
  memory impairment/loss
  reaction time impairment
  psychological impairment

Dependence/independence in maintaining a safe environment
  mental problems
  physical problems

PLANNING

IMPLEMENTATION
of nursing activities such as

Orientating patient to new physical environment

Matching of bed/chair to patient

Maintaining a quiet environment

Helping to decrease patients' anxiety

Liaising with domestic staff to maintain hygiene standards

Practising/facilitating/encouraging handwashing

Teaching patients and public about maintaining a safe environment

Giving medications safely/keeping drugs safely

Helping impaired patients to maintain a safe environment

EVALUATION

Communicating

ASSESSMENT

Influencing factors
  stage of development
  physical factors
    speaking
    seeing
    hearing
    reading
    writing
  psychological factors
    level of intelligence
    extent of vocabulary
    nervousness
    prevailing mood
    level of self-respect
  sociocultural factors
    native language
    local vocabulary
    accent/dialect
    personal appearance/dress
    touching
    eye-contact
    gesticulation
  environmental factors
    response to:
        type/size of room
        arrangement of chairs
        background noise
        light
        room temperature
    individual habit

Visual perception

Aural perception

Congruence of body and verbal language

Orientation
  time of day
  day of week
  month of year

ANALYSIS OF DATA

IDENTIFICATION OF PATIENTS' PROBLEMS

Change of environment
  unfamiliar people
  unfamiliar place
  unfamiliar language
  unfamiliar activities
  change of status and roles

Change in mode of communicating
  impaired cognition
  impaired/loss of sight
  impaired/loss of hearing
  impaired/loss of sensation
  impaired/loss of mobility
  impaired/loss of speech

Dependence/independence in communicating
  cognitive problems
  speaking problems
  hearing problems
  reading and writing problems
  body language problems

Discomforts associated with communicating
  pain
  social embarrassment

PLANNING

IMPLEMENTATION
of nursing activities such as

Introducing patients to nurses and other patients

Talking with a purpose to patients and others

Establishing/maintaining/terminating nurse-patient relationships satisfactorily

Giving information clearly to patients and others

Teaching patients and others

Keeping patients orientated in time and place

Helping to prevent patients from feeling stigmatised

Communicating with:
    deaf and hard of hearing patients
    blind and visually-impaired patients
    speech-impaired patients
    cognitively-impaired patients
    illiterate patients
    immobile patients
    breathless patients

Easing difficulty with speaking

Easing difficulty with seeing

Easing difficulty with hearing

Alleviating pain interfering with communicating

EVALUATION

Breathing

ASSESSMENT

Respiration and relationship to
   age
   weight
   pulse rate
   body temperature
   activity level
   emotional status
   colour of:
      skin
      mucous membrane
      nail bed

Character of breathing
   rate
   depth
   rhythm
   sound

Difficulty associated with breathing
   on inspiration/expiration
   on lying down
   on exertion

Cough (if present)
   when it occurs
   frequency
   what relieves it
   relationship to smoking
   sputum:
      amount
      colour
      odour

Smoking habits (if acquired)
   type of smoking:
      cigarette
      cigar
      pipe
   frequency
   tar content of tobacco
   reason for smoking
   intention to continue/give up
   relationship to present illness
   knowledge about adverse effects

Exposure to/knowledge of air pollution
   at home
   at work
   in neighbourhood

ANALYSIS OF DATA

IDENTIFICATION OF PATIENTS' PROBLEMS

Change of environment and routine

Change in breathing habit
   upper respiratory tract congestion
   excessive secretions
   bronchial spasms
   dyspnoea:
      interference with:
         speaking
         eating
         drinking
         working and playing
         mobilising
         sleeping
         expressing sexuality

Dependence/independence in breathing
   obstructed air passages
   oxygen insufficiency
   mechanical defect
   respiratory failure

Discomforts associated with breathing
   cough
   sputum
   haemoptysis
   allergy
   pain
   anxiety

Presence of
   artificial airway
   tracheostomy
   artificial ventilation equipment

Inability to give up/reduce smoking

PLANNING

IMPLEMENTATION
of nursing activities such as

Allaying anxiety associated with dyspnoea

Relieving dyspnoea

Administering oxygen

Maintaining an artificial airway

Maintaining tracheostomy toilet

Helping patient to expectorate sputum

Preventing/counteracting respiratory failure

Teaching and helping with breathing exercises

Alleviating discomforts associated with breathing

Assessing pain associated with breathing

Providing health education about:
   smoking
   room ventilation
   air pollution

EVALUATION

Eating and drinking

ASSESSMENT

Influencing factors
- age and sex
- height and weight
- occupation and activity
- state of mouth and teeth
- proficiency in taking food and drink
- emotional status
- family traditions
- sociocultural idiosyncrasies
- religious commendations/
  restrictions
- finance available for food/drink
- physical environment

Individual habits
- timing and location of meals
- quantity and quality of diet
- consumption of alcohol
- dietary likes and dislikes
- deliberate restrictions/indulgences
- company at mealtimes

Knowledge about/attitudes to
- the effect of diet on health
- obesity
- alcoholism
- food hygiene
- disposal of food waste

Ability to procure food and fluid
- facilities for growing food/procuring
  water
- choice and price of food/fluid
- distance from home to shopping area
- availability of transport
- ability to carry shopping

Storage and cooking facilities
- means of storage
- means of cooking

Aids needed for independence
- special utensils
- mechanical aids
- kitchen gadgets
- special transport for shopping

Appetite for food/fluid

Pain associated with eating and drinking
- location/severity
- type/duration

Discomforts
- nausea/vomiting
- indigestion/flatulence

ANALYSIS OF DATA

IDENTIFICATION OF PATIENTS' PROBLEMS

Change of environment and routine
- timing of meals
- serving of meals
- pre- and post-meal activities
- alteration in appetite
- separation from mother

Dependence/independence
- problems associated with physical
  dependence
- problems associated with emotional
  dependence

Change in eating and drinking habits
- modification of habitual food intake
- modification of habitual fluid intake

Change in mode of eating and drinking
- nasogastric feeding
- gastrostomy feeding
- intravenous feeding

Discomforts associated with eating and drinking
- stomatitis
- nausea
- vomiting
- heartburn
- flatulence
- halitosis
- pain
- anxiety about investigations

PLANNING

IMPLEMENTATION
of nursing activities such as

Providing assistance necessary for
procuring/preparing food

Providing assistance/special
equipment necessary for eating and
drinking

Feeding by artificial routes

Maintaining an intravenous infusion

Assisting with planning and preparing
special diets

Teaching about special diets

Monitoring and recording food/fluid
intake

Preventing and controlling dehydration
and oedema

Assessing/alleviating pain associated
with eating/drinking

Alleviating discomforts associated with
eating/drinking

Providing health education about
nutrition and alcoholism

Controlling environmental factors
which affect preparation/eating/
disposal of foods and fluids

EVALUATION

Eliminating

ASSESSMENT

Urinary elimination
  micturition frequency
  urine output/fluid balance
  appearance, smell, composition of
    urine
  discomforts associated with
    micturition

Faecal elimination
  defaecation frequency
  factors altering frequency of
    defaecation
  amount, appearance, composition of
    faeces
  dietary habits, including fibre intake
  measures taken to prevent
    constipation
  discomforts associated with
    defaecation

Personal eliminating routine/habits
  usual daily eliminating routine
  type of toilet facilities available in
    ward/home/work
  habits regarding perineal toilet
  habits regarding handwashing after
    eliminating

**Dependence/independence in
eliminating**
  degree of independence in
    eliminating, related to age,
    physical/mental/health
    status, available toilet facilities
  use of/need for special equipment/
    appliances
  history and nature of incontinence, if
    relevant
  details of catheter/stoma
    management, if relevant

ANALYSIS OF DATA

IDENTIFICATION OF PATIENTS' PROBLEMS

Change of environment and routine
  unfamiliar environment of hospital
  unfamiliar routine of hospital life
  lack of privacy in the ward

**Dependence/independence in
eliminating**
  dependence due to:
    limited mobility
    confinement to bed
    psychological disturbance

Change in urine and its elimination
  anxiety about change in appearance
    of urine
  increased frequency of micturition
  increased/decreased output of
    urine
  urinary incontinence
  urinary catheterisation

Change in faeces and their elimination
  anxiety about change in appearance
    of faeces
  increased frequency of defaecation:
    diarrhoea
  decreased frequency of defaecation:
    constipation
  inability to defaecate: impaction
  faecal incontinence
  ileostomy/colostomy

**Discomforts associated with
eliminating**
  pain associated with micturition
  pain associated with defaecation
  anxiety associated with related
    investigations

PLANNING

IMPLEMENTATION
of nursing activities such as

Providing opportunities, facilities,
  privacy for eliminating

Giving assistance to dependent patients

Practising/facilitating/encouraging
  handwashing

Ensuring safe disposal of excreta

Collecting and testing specimens of
  urine/faeces

Monitoring and recording fluid balance

Catheterisation and catheter care

Preventing and treating constipation/
  faecal impaction

Nursing a patient with diarrhoea

Nursing a patient with a stoma

Alleviating and preventing discomforts
  associated with eliminating

Assessing and alleviating pain
  associated with eliminating

Preparation of patients undergoing
  investigations

Assisting/retraining the incontinent
  patient

Teaching people about the AL of
  eliminating

Teaching people how to prevent and
  recognise related problems

EVALUATION

Personal cleansing and dressing

ASSESSMENT

Influencing factors
 sex and stage of development
 environment: fixed bath/shower;
  piped hot/cold water
 economic status; occupation climate;
  cultural attitudes
 individual habit

Skin
 appearance: colour/bruising/scars;
  turgid/wrinkled; dry/moist;
  blemishes
 areas of discontinuity: maceration;
  athlete's foot; skin lesion/disease;
  incision; pressure sores
 degree of risk of pressure sores
 bathing/showering: frequency; time
  of day; aids needed/help required

Hands and nails
 cleanliness; condition; abnormalities
 evidence of type of occupation
 handwashing routine/facilities

Hair
 style, length, type: dry/greasy; dull/
  shiny
 presence of dandruff/nits
 baldness
 relationship to diet and health
 hair washing routine/help required

Mouth and teeth
 moistness/dryness of mouth/tongue
  /lips
 odour of breath
 teeth: appearance; presence/
  absence; plate, dentures/help
  required; cleaning routine/help
  required

Dress
 style/colour/fashion
 quality/newness of garments
 quality/suitability of footwear
 standard of cleanliness/odour
 special clothing

Dressing
 mobility problems
 necessary modifications/help needed

ANALYSIS OF DATA

IDENTIFICATION OF PATIENTS' PROBLEMS

Change of environment and routine
 unfamiliar ward routine
 interference with daily routine
 lessened decision making
 lack of privacy

Change in mode of personal cleansing and dressing
 imposed non-bathing
 modification of clothing
 wearing a prosthesis

Dependence/independence in personal cleansing and dressing
 limited mobility
 absence of limbs
 involuntary movements
 sensory deficits
 unconsciousness
 psychological disturbance
 illness

Loss of skin continuity
 incision
 trauma
 skin disease
 pressure sores

Discomforts associated with personal cleansing and dressing
 psychological discomfort
 increased sweating

PLANNING

IMPLEMENTATION
of nursing activities such as

Providing opportunities, facilities, privacy for continuance of patients' individual habits

Giving assistance to dependent patients without loss of their dignity

Providing opportunity for patients to make decisions about their personal cleansing and dressing

Using resources to help patients select modified clothing and aids to independence

Teaching patients and the public about personal hygiene by, among other methods, acting as a role model

Preparing patients' skin for operation

Carrying out wound dressing procedures with aseptic technique

Monitoring patients at risk of developing pressure sores

Preventing and treating pressure sores

Treating infested patients

Helping patients who have an itching skin

EVALUATION

Controlling body temperature

ASSESSMENT

Measurement of body temperature
changes in body temperature over
time
relationship of ascertained
temperature and changes to
physiological, emotional,
environmental and socio-
economic factors
ability to assist in controlling body
temperature
subjective feeling of being too
warm/cold

**Indicators of an abnormally high
temperature**
flushed skin
increased sweating
increased pulse rate
decreased urine output
anorexia
disorientation

**Indicators of an abnormally low
temperature**
pallor
shivering
decreased respiration rate/pulse/
BP
lethargy
impairment of consciousness

Risk of developing hypothermia

**Knowledge of causes/prevention/
treatment of**
pyrexia
heatstroke
hypothermia

ANALYSIS OF DATA

IDENTIFICATION OF PATIENTS' PROBLEMS

Uncomfortable environmental
temperature

Abnormally high body temperature

Abnormally low body temperature

PLANNING

IMPLEMENTATION
of nursing activities such as

Regulating environmental temperature

Measuring/recording body
temperature

For a pyrexial patient
preventing further increase of body
temperature
reducing body temperature to
patient's normal level
alleviating discomforts associated

For a hypothermic patient
restoring body temperature to
patient's normal level
maintaining vital functions of the
body

Prevention and early detection of
hypothermia

Prevention of illness due to heat

EVALUATION

Mobilising

ASSESSMENT

Influencing factors
developmental
physical
psychological
environmental
social

Mobilising habits
at home/work/play

Musculoskeletal status
adequacy of nervous and
  cardiopulmonary systems
body posture and gait
muscle strength, mass, tone
range of movement in limbs, trunk,
  head and neck
range of facial mobility
joint movement and related stiffness/
  pain

**Dependence/independence in
mobilising**
level of independence in the AL of
  mobilising
mode of transport to work/school/
  shops
aids needed for independent
  mobilising
factors limiting independence

Knowledge and attitudes
knowledge about the body's exercise
  needs
attitude to physical handicap

ANALYSIS OF DATA

IDENTIFICATION OF PATIENTS' PROBLEMS

Change in mobilising routine

**Lack of specific knowledge about
mobilising routine**

Change in mobilising habit
restricted mobility, including bedrest
impairment of body or limb
  movement
hyperactivity/hypoactivity
physical handicap

Dependence in mobilising
upper limb defect
lower limb defect

Discomforts
musculoskeletal discomforts
therapeutic immobilising
  procedures
pain
social/economic and emotional
  discomforts

PLANNING

IMPLEMENTATION
of nursing activities such as

Giving assistance to patients with
  restricted mobility

Preventing/alleviating discomforts
  associated with reduced mobility

Assessing and alleviating pain
  associated with mobilising

Helping patients to accept and cope with
  the physical, socio-economic and
  psychological problems arising from
  restricted mobility

Lifting and moving patients

Teaching/supervising deep breathing
  exercises

Assisting with passive/active exercises

Providing/assisting with use of special
  equipment to aid mobilising

Restructuring the environment to
  maximise independence

Assisting/protecting the hyperactive/
  hypoactive patient

Planning, implementing and evaluating
  rehabilitation related to mobilising

Educating the public about physical
  handicap: implications/prevention

Educating the public about the body's
  exercise needs

Teaching people safe lifting techniques

EVALUATION

Working and playing

ASSESSMENT

Influencing factors
   physical factors:
      ability/disability
   communicating ability
   psychological factors:
      intelligence
      motivation
      temperament and personality
         traits
   cultural and religious factors
   climatic and environmental factors
   economic factors

Routine regarding
   time spent working/playing
   place of working/playing
   travel to place of working/playing
   safety while working/playing
   holidays from work/date of last one

Attitudes and habits regarding
   punctuality and self-discipline
   reliability and honesty
   fulfilment/boredom
   colleagues at work and play
   sharing in group activities
   earning and spending money

**Relationship between working/
playing and**
   age and sex
   emotional status
   family circumstances
   socio-economic status

Health status
   effect of present illness on working/
      playing

**Aids needed for independence in
working/playing**
   special transport
   special equipment

Knowledge and attitudes to
   sick-leave from work
   sickness benefit
   safety at work /play
   the importance of playing

ANALYSIS OF DATA

IDENTIFICATION OF PATIENTS' PROBLEMS

Change of environment and routine
   change of working and playing
      routines
   absence from family groups
   absence from work and play groups

**Dependence/independence in
working and playing**
   congenital mental and/or physical
      handicap
   chronic disabling disease
   impairment of the nervous system
   mental illness
   frailty

Change in working and playing habits
   sensory deficits
   physical disablement
   physical disfigurement
   change due to drug taking

**Discomforts associated with working
and playing**
   boredom
   lack of fresh air and exercise
   economic hardship

PLANNING

IMPLEMENTATION
of nursing activities such as

Preventing boredom/providing
stimulation
   playing/talking with patients
   discussing with patient/parent/
      guardian :
         visiting/visitors
         rooming-in
         how the patients will occupy
            themselves
   enabling patients' activities to fit in to
      treatment programme
   helping patients to continue their
      health habits/walking outside

Preventing loneliness
   helping patients to benefit from
      visitors
   introducing patients to those with
      similiar interests

Procuring aids to independence

Co-ordinating the contribution of:
   occupational health service
   Disablement Resettlement Officer
   physiotherapists
   occupational therapists
   industrial therapists
   speech therapists
   social workers

Helping patients to return to, or change,
their working/playing habits

Helping patients with financial problems

EVALUATION

Expressing sexuality

ASSESSMENT

Stage of sexual development

Mode of expressing sexuality
    in appearance, general behaviour,
    communication

Influencing factors
    gender
    stage of development
    nature of relationship network
    personal preference
    social and family background

Effects of hospitalisation/disease/ disability
    on sexual development
    sexual relationships
    sexual function
    mode of expressing sexuality

Knowledge and attitudes about sex and reproduction
    if relevant, history related to
    menstruation, contraception,
    pregnancy and parity
    if relevant, detailed assessment of
    discomforts/dysfunction
    related to sexual organs/
    function

ANALYSIS OF DATA

IDENTIFICATION OF PATIENTS' PROBLEMS

Anxiety/embarrassment about
    intimate procedures

Lack of privacy in the hospital ward

Restrictions on normal sexual
    development/activity imposed by
    hospitalisation

Sexual difficulties arising from
    physical disease
    physical disability
    physical disfigurement

PLANNING

IMPLEMENTATION
of nursing activities such as

Preventing embarrassment/anxiety
    over intimate procedures

Providing maximum privacy for patients

Minimising disruption to established
    sexual habits/relationships during
    illness/hospitalisation

Ensuring opportunities for normal
    sexual development during long-
    term hospitalisation

Providing information about resuming/
    restricting sexual activity after
    illness or surgery

Helping patients to cope with sexual
    difficulties

Preventing/alleviating discomforts
    associated with sexual function

Helping people to understand, develop
    and enjoy their sexuality

Health education about sex,
    reproduction, contraception, sexually
    transmitted diseases, sexual
    difficulties

EVALUATION

Sleeping

ASSESSMENT

Usual sleeping environment
  bed/bedding/personal night attire
  own/shared bed
  own/shared bedroom
  noise/quietness
  hot/cold

Usual sleeping behaviour
  work-shift/sleep pattern
  time of going to bed
  time of going to sleep
  wakening during sleep/time of such
    waking
  movement during sleep
  snoring
  time of wakening at end of sleep
    period
  time of rising

**Patient's estimation of usual
sleeping**
  good/bad sleeper
  refreshed/unrefreshed on waking
  mood on rising

Other factors influencing sleep
  biological clock
  daytime exercise
  sleeping pills

Factors interfering with sleep
  mood
  worry, anxiety, apprehension
  boredom
  pain

Level of consciousness

ANALYSIS OF DATA

IDENTIFICATION OF PATIENTS' PROBLEMS

Change of environment and routine
  bed, bedding, night attire
  pre-sleep routine
  posture
  environmental temperature
  noise
  light
  disturbance of circadian rhythm

Discomforts associated with sleeping
  insomnia
    inability to get to sleep
    excessive wakefulness
    early morning waking
  restlessness
  cramp
  pain

Impairment of consciousness
  coma
  convulsions

PLANNING

IMPLEMENTATION
of nursing activities such as

Facilitating continuation of pre-sleep
  routines

Ensuring comfortable environment for
  sleeping

Monitoring/recording sufficient/
  insufficient sleep

Preventing/alleviating factors
  interfering with sleep

Assessing and alleviating pain

Helping people to understand their sleep
  needs

Helping patients to cope with worries
  about sleeping

Safe administration, and monitoring
  effectiveness of sleeping pills

Health education about the hazards of
  sleeping pills

Care of an anaesthetised patient

Care of a comatose patient

Care of a convulsing patient

EVALUATION

Dying

ASSESSMENT

The person's
physical status
degree of pain
discomforts
degree of dependence/
independence in all ALs
awareness of the prognosis
mood and behaviour
fears and anxieties
religion/beliefs about death and
dying
family and social circumstances
wishes regarding care during
terminal illness (including place
of care, treatments, contact with
family/others/chaplain)

The family's (significant others)
knowledge of the prognosis
understanding the implications of
the prognosis
reactions to this knowledge
wishes regarding management of
the terminal illness
wish to contribute to care
need for emotional support
need for preparation for
bereavement
need for support in bereavement

ANALYSIS OF DATA

IDENTIFICATION OF PATIENTS' PROBLEMS

Physical problems associated with terminal illness
pain
other physical discomforts

Psychological problems in the terminal illness
patient's problems
relatives' problems

Problems associated with bereavement
physical problems
emotional problems

PLANNING

IMPLEMENTATION
of nursing activities such as

Helping the patient to die with dignity

Preventing suffering from pain in the terminal illness

Alleviating discomforts associated with all ALs

Providing companionship/preventing loneliness

Listening to anxieties/allaying fears and anxieties

Respecting as far as possible the patient's wishes

Providing opportunities and privacy for contact with loved ones

Providing information for relatives/visitors

Providing emotional support for relatives/visitors

Preparing relatives for bereavement

Providing support for colleagues

Educating people about death, dying and bereavement

EVALUATION

3

Assessing patients

In the Introduction, the assessment phase of the process of nursing was described and guidelines given about how to collect patient data from assessment.

A common criticism made of the nursing process is that nurses just do not have time to make and document nursing assessments of all patients. It is interesting to note, as Kratz (1979) points out:

> ... doctors, irrespective of how busy they may be, always find time to record a new patient's medical history. Nursing process requires that nurses place equal importance on the collection of nursing information as do doctors on collecting medical information.

In fact, with the help of an appropriate nursing assessment form and a nursing framework within which to assess patients, once practised in the art of collecting relevant data, making and documenting assessments of patients need not be excessively time-consuming. And it is a necessary prerequisite of planning, implementing and evaluating a patient's nursing.

Different aspects of assessment, using the Patient Assessment Form already described (pp. 7–10), are illustrated in this section by three patients.

Firstly, *assessing a patient on admission* to hospital is illustrated by the first two patients described: a middle-aged man admitted for investigation of haematuria and a little girl admitted to a children's ward with burns due to an accident at home.

Secondly, the *essential ongoing nature of assessing patients* is illustrated in the case of an elderly man who lives at home and who is under the supervision of a health visitor.

Readers are referred to the summary charts of the twelve ALs (pp 11–22) in each of which, under the column headed 'assessment' is listed relevant points to bear in mind when assessing each activity of living. Some guidelines have already been given in the Introduction on assessing the various ALs (pp 1–4).

MR GORDON MITCHELL Age 48
Admitted for investigation of haematuria

Several times in recent weeks, Mr Mitchell a 48-year-old architect, had passed urine with blood in it (haematuria). Although he felt concerned about this—and, in fact, had been considerably alarmed the first time—it was only when he began to experience some discomfort while passing urine that he decided to go to his doctor.

The GP explained to Mr Mitchell that it was important for the cause of his symptoms to be investigated without delay. So, within the week, Mr Mitchell was admitted to the genito-urinary ward for cystoscopy and biopsy.

PREPARING FOR 'THE ADMISSION ASSESSMENT'

Information which the nurse has in advance of the patient's arrival in the ward can be used in preparation for the assessment. Knowing as she does the reason for this patient's admission and his age, the nurse can assume that Mr Mitchell will be able to cope with, and will appreciate the necessity for, an admission interview. If she knows nothing of the patient's socio-economic and ethnic background, the nurse must be ready to adjust the type and degree of difficulty of her questions according to her immediate assessment of the patient's circumstances and intellectual ability. Being an architect, it can be assumed that Mr Mitchell will have no difficulty in understanding and answering the nurse's questions.

However, he may experience discomfort and perhaps embarrassment at being asked personal questions by the nurse. Such discomfort may result from role reversal, Mr Mitchell finding himself in a submissive role when usually

23

at work he plays the dominant role. Or else, his embarrassment may derive from his being asked questions about usually private activities by a nurse, perhaps young enough to be his daughter. Being aware of the various feelings patients may experience during this 'routine' admission assessment will guide the nurse towards sensitive questioning and establishing rapport with the patient.

Sometimes, as in this case, knowing the reason for the patient's admission can be very important. Although haematuria is a symptom of many kinds of urinary system disorders, painless haematuria (which Mr Mitchell experienced initially) is the first symptom in the majority of bladder tumours. This is why early investigation is advised by doctors. Even if Mr Mitchell has no idea that his symptom could conceivably suggest cancer, he probably realises that it may suggest a serious condition on account of the speed with which his admission was arranged.

The nurse, in any case, should be aware that the patient is likely to be anxious during the assessment interview and she should attempt to minimise anxiety.

A further consideration of this patient's reason for admission is the fact that he is being admitted for investigation (rather than for treatment, at least in the first instance) and, in particular, for the investigation named 'cystoscopy and biopsy'. This involves inspection of the interior of the bladder by means of an endoscope introduced through the urethra. It is usually performed under anaesthetic. Thus, the nurse should be aware that the patient is being admitted specifically for an investigation which, in this case, involves a general anaesthetic. These facts should help to direct the nurse's questioning and, in particular, to indicate less and more relevant aspects to be assessed in relation to the patient's activities of living.

COLLECTING BIOGRAPHICAL/HEALTH DATA

The left-hand side of the Patient Assessment Form (p. 26) is concerned with biographical and health data. Much of this may be completed, prior to the patient's arrival, from his previous health records or information already received in the ward. It is tedious for the patient to be asked to provide these details time and time again—in the reception or casualty department, by the nurses, the doctors—but the nurse must check with the patient that the details she has are correct.

In Mr Mitchell's case, his *surname* and *forenames, age, address* and *reason for admission* could be inserted on his Patient Assessment Form (Fig. 3.1) in readiness for his admission interview. Unless it is obvious, it is necessary to ask how the patient *prefers to be addressed*. The gender (*male/female*) should be noted on the form and whether or not the patient is *single/married/widowed*. This information provides the staff with knowledge which may influence, for example, their conversation with the patient and whether

or not there is a spouse to consider when planning the patient's nursing. In addition, asking about marital status will provide information about recent change in status. Getting married or divorced, or suffering bereavement, are *significant life crises*. It is known that illness can be related to such life crises and it is inevitable that they will influence the patient's relationships in hospital and his attitude to his illness and rehabilitation.

Mr Mitchell's personal circumstances turned out to be rather complicated. He explained that he had recently separated from his wife (this fact entered on the form against 'other'), although her name (with address) was given as *next of kin*, which is a legal relationship. However, Mr Mitchell was anxious that she was not contacted without his permission. When asked about *significant others* Mr Mitchell said that he had two grown-up sons but, as both lived elsewhere, he had not informed them of his admission. He had told his business partner about his admission to hospital and gave this person's name as the only visitor he expected during what he anticipated would be a very brief stay in hospital. When a patient's personal circumstances are as complicated as this, it might seem to be none of a nurse's business. But nowadays, when separation and divorce are common, it is important to be aware of the various possible circumstances. Knowing about a patient's circumstances should help nurses to avoid tactless conversation, understand who for that patient are 'significant others', and identify possible problems in respect of visiting and eventual discharge.

Address of normal residence which, in Mr Mitchell's case was also his work address, is recorded in full on the form. Details of the *type of accommodation* were not relevant here. The fact that Mr Mitchell lives alone is recorded alongside *family/others at this residence*.

An architect by *occupation*, Mr Mitchell's brief admission to hospital is unlikely to cause much disruption at work. However, he can be expected to feel anxious about whether his symptom of haematuria could indicate an illness requiring treatment in hospital, which might necessitate time away from running his business.

It is always necessary to know of any *religious beliefs and practices* which may affect the patient's nursing, or his attitude to his illness and treatment. The fact that Mr Mitchell is Roman Catholic is noted on the assessment form for future reference.

To allow the patient an opportunity to relax at the admission interview and perhaps to offer unsolicited, but relevant, information, the nurse can encourage him to talk about his *perception of current health status*, his understanding of the reason for *admission/referral*, what he knows of the *medical diagnosis* and of his *past medical history*. Any known *allergies* should also be recorded. The nurse can then compare the patient's understanding of his present and past health status with the information in the medical notes. She may discover from this that he is well informed—as Mr Mitchell was of his particular circumstances—or, alternatively, that he is poorly informed or misinformed. In the latter circumstances, the nurse can then act to rectify the position.

COLLECTING DATA ABOUT ALs

Data collected about Mr Mitchell's ALs are summarised on the right-hand side of his Patient Assessment Form (Fig. 3.1). The patient's health problem (haematuria) did not involve debilitation and therefore, as could be expected of this adult, educated patient he was found to be independent in all ALs. Therefore, only minimal essential data need be written on the form and, when collecting it, the nurse would have in mind two points: firstly, that Mr Mitchell was being admitted specifically for an investigation and, therefore, may not stay in hospital for more than a day or two and, secondly, that the scheduled investigation could involve a general anaesthetic. Thus, only data necessary for short-term planning and preparation for anaesthesia were required in relation to assessment of Mr Mitchell's ALs. In contrast, in the next patient presentation the need for very detailed data on all ALs is shown, the patient being a highly dependent child.

JANE THOMSON   Age 21 months

Admitted with burns

It was late one Saturday evening when Jane Thomson was admitted as an 'emergency admission' to the waiting children's ward, after an accident at home.

While Mrs Thomson was feeding the baby and Mr Thomson was watching television, Jane had wandered into the kitchenette. Standing on tiptoe, she had pulled off from the gas cooker the saucepan which contained the remainder of the water just boiled to heat her baby brother's feed. The hot water had splashed on to the side of her neck and run down her chest and partly over her right arm.

While Mrs Thomson attended to her screaming daughter her husband rushed next door to use a neighbour's phone to ring for an ambulance. Jane was still crying when, quarter of an hour later, her father carried her from the ambulance into the casualty department of the children's hospital.

There Jane's clothing was carefully removed and she was given by injection an analgesic drug. Once transferred to the ward, the burned areas of her skin were cleaned and, on the doctor's advice dressings were applied. These were covered with padded splints secured by bandages in order to prevent Jane from scratching or knocking the burns. Throughout this procedure, the nurses did all they could to console Jane and her very distressed father.

Jane was now ready to be carried by a nurse to an individual cubicle which had been prepared, where the doctor joined them to check Jane's condition once more and write on her medication chart a prescription of a sedative drug to be given later that night. Meanwhile Jane's father was helped into a gown and he willingly agreed to the suggestion that he sit beside the cot for a while, in the hope that Jane would soon fall asleep. In fact, Jane, exhausted by the events of the evening, was asleep within a very short time.

Mr Thomson was told that he could stay overnight in the hospital. However, he explained that not having a phone he had no way of contacting his wife to give her news of Jane, and so he decided to go home. The nurse reassured him that Jane would be carefully looked after and acknowledged she understood how difficult it must have been for Jane's mother to accept that she had to stay at home with the baby while Jane's father took Jane to the hospital.

Before leaving, however, Mr Thomson agreed to give the nurse-in-charge any information about Jane that was required. The nurse thanked Mr Thomson for his cooperation, and assured him it would not take long, as she appreciated he was keen to get home to give his wife news of Jane.

COLLECTING BIOGRAPHICAL/HEALTH DATA

The nurse already knew, from the admission form made out in the casualty department, Jane's full *name*, her *age* and *address* and the fact that Mr Thomson as Jane's father, was her *next of kin*. The fact that the patient was habitually *addressed as* Jane, rather than by any pet name, was confirmed.

Next, remembering that the home is without a phone, the nurse asked if there was any neighbour or near relative who could be telephoned if Jane's parents needed to be contacted urgently. The name and the *phone number* of the next door neighbour were ascertained. Mr Thomson suggested that his mother-in-law who lives near them could take a phone message any weekday morning at the house where she is employed as a home-help. This relative, Jane's grandmother, would be referred as one of Jane's *significant others*, along with her mother and father, baby brother and maternal grandfather. (Paternal grandparents live in another city).

The nurse discovered when discussing possible visiting arrangements that Mr Thomson was, by *occupation*, a factory worker but that he is currently unemployed. Mrs Thomson has never worked outside the home. He was asked if the staff needed to know of any *religious beliefs and*

Patient Assessment Form

Date of admission   *6 May*   Date of assessment   *6 May*

Surname   *MITCHELL*   Forenames   *Gordon Peter*

Male ☑   Age *48*   ~~Single~~/Married/~~Widowed~~
Female ☐   Date of birth   Other *but separated from wife*

Prefers to be addressed as   *Mr Mitchell*

Address of usual residence   *13 High Street Newtown*

Type of accommodation   *Flat above business premises*

Family/Others at this residence   *Lives alone*

Next of kin ✱   Name   *Anne Mitchell*   Address   *4 Hillview Crescent Newtown*
Relationship   *Wife (separated)*   Tel. no.   *—*

✱ Not inform[ed] of admission to be contacte[d] without patie[nt] permission.

Significant others   Relatives/~~Dependents~~   *2 adult sons (neither informed of admission)*

Helpers   *———*

Visitors   *No family visitors. Partner (J. Davey) may visit.*

Occupation   *Architect: own business with one partner.*

Religious beliefs and relevant practices   *Roman Catholic*

Patient's perception of current health status   *Understands that haematuria indicates some dysfunction of the urinary system and requires investigation.*

Reason for admission/~~referral~~   *Investigation of haematuria: cystoscopy and biopsy*

Medical diagnosis   *None, as yet*

Past medical history   *Appendix removed at age 17*

Allergies   *None*

Significant life crises   *Recently separated from wife*

Fig. 3.1 Mr Mitchell: assessment of ALs

Assessment of Activities of Living

Date **6 May**

AL	Usual routines: what he/she can and cannot do independently	Patient's problems (actual/potential) (p) = potential

● Maintaining a safe environment

Independent

● Communicating

Fluent, articulate in speech. Communicates with ease. Conveys anxiety about forthcoming investigation / possible causes of haematuria.

● Breathing

Smokes 15 cigarettes per day. Has a productive morning cough. Does not become breathless on exertion.

● Eating and drinking

Good appetite. Is not overweight. Prefers natural foodstuffs. Dislikes fish and eggs. Does not drink alcohol in excess.

● Eliminating

Apart from recent onset of haematuria and dysuria, micturition is normal. Bowels regular (daily).

● Personal cleansing and dressing

Meticulous standard of cleanliness and grooming. Showers and shaves daily (a.m.) Wears full dentures.

● Controlling body temperature

Body temperature within range of normal on admission.

● Mobilising

Full range of movement. Very active. Jogs daily; swims regularly.

● Working and playing

Business (architecture) is main activity and interest in life, especially since recent separation from wife. Plays squash weekly.

● Expressing sexuality

Nil of note.

● Sleeping

Good sleeper; retires at 2330 hrs, rises at 0600 hrs. Does not take sleeping tablets.

● Dying

Patient Assessment Form

Date of admission   *10 November*   Date of assessment   *10 November*

Surname   **THOMSON**   Forenames   *Jane*

Male ☐
Female ☑

Age / Date of birth   *21/12*

Single/Married/Widowed
Other

Prefers to be addressed as   *Jane*

Address of usual residence   *213 Bridge Road, Billington.*

Type of accommodation   *Small flat; shared w.c.; no bath / hot water supply.*

Family/~~Others~~ at this residence   *Parents and baby brother.*

Next of kin   Name   *John Thomson*   Address   *as above.*

Relationship   *Father*   Tel. no. *{ of neighbour (Mrs Brown) 022-73231*
{ of grandmother's work (a.m.) 022-84

Significant others   Relatives/~~Dependents~~   *Parents. Baby brother (4 months) - Michael*

Helpers

Visitors   *Maternal grandparents*

Occupation   *(Father's) Unemployed factory worker*

Religious beliefs and relevant practices   *No religion*

Patient's perception of current health status

Reason for admission/~~referral~~   *Burns from scalding accident at home.*

Medical diagnosis   *Superficial burns: part neck, chest, R arm.*

Past medical history   *Frequent colds. No serious illness / no previous hospital admission.*

Allergies   *None.*   Significant life crises

Fig. 3.2 Jane Thomson: assessment of ALs

Assessment of Activities of Living

Date *10/11 Nov.*

AL	Usual routines: what he/she can and cannot do independently	Patient's problems (actual/potential) (p) = potential

● Maintaining a safe environment

Dependent on others for safety. Does respond to 'No!' and 'Stop that!' Currently prone to accidents / falls when imitating adults' activities.

● Communicating

Has started to speak; single words (Mummy, Daddy, baby, bed, juice, no, kisses, "Letty" = Lamb, potty). Understands / responds to simple phrases.

● Breathing

Constantly runny nose; frequent colds. Respirations 35/minute on admission: pulse 128/min

● Eating and drinking

'Good eater'; able to spoonfeed self. Juice at 0630; breakfast - cereal; lunch at 1200, (eg. sausages); tea at 1700; milk before bed. Prefers juice to milk / sweet foods to savoury. Reluctant to drink since admission.

● Eliminating

In nappies at all times. Uses potty after meals. B.O. after breakfast / tea. Stools sometimes loose. Refers to stools and urine as "pee". Strong-smelling nappy this a.m.

● Personal cleansing and dressing

Used to twice weekly 'bath' in sink / weekly hairwash. Observed to have dirty, ragged nails. Does not clean teeth. Likes to help wash / dress self.

● Controlling body temperature

Temperature at 2200 hrs Saturday (10/10)   38·2°C
0600 hrs Sunday (11/10)   37·8°C
1000 hrs Sunday (11/10)   38·0°C
Flushed and hot on waking this a.m.

● Mobilising

Active child. Full range of movement. Has recently learned to walk downstairs, holding rail.

● Working and playing

Plays well by self. Favourite toys 'playpeople', books, dolls, saucepan set, toy lamb ("Letty"). Loves being read to (especially nursery rhymes).

● Expressing sexuality

Parents anxious about possibility of permanent disfigurement from burns.

● Sleeping

'Bad sleeper.' Cries at bedtime (1700-2100 hrs); wakes crying, approx 0400. Wakens about 0630. Sleeps in cot in room with rest of family. No pillow; sleepsuit and 2 blankets.

● Dying

practices and replied that none of the family belonged to any church.

Information about the *type of accommodation* had already been elicited in the course of earlier conversation. Mr Thomson had mentioned that Jane's accident had been caused, in part at least, by their overcrowded conditions. They lived in a small tenement flat comprising a tiny kitchenette and two rooms; the toilet was out on the landing and shared with others. Even this basic information about Jane's home conditions was sufficient to make the nurse wonder how the parents might be helped to improve safety standards in their home.

There was minimal information to record about Jane's *past medical history*. Her father said she often had colds but apart from that was healthy. As far as he was aware, she had had no problems as a baby. It seemed that Jane's mother had not had her immunised at all. Recently the health visitor had called to try to persuade them to take the new baby to the clinic for his first immunisation, but had been unsuccessful.

These pieces of information, obtained in a relatively brief interview with Jane's father, provided basic and essential data about the patient. Readers will recognise these data in summary form on the left-hand side of the Patient Assessment Form (Fig. 3.2, p. 28). Also entered is the *reason for admission* and the *medical diagnosis*.

COLLECTING DATA ABOUT ALs

Even although it was clear that Jane's parents would be able, between them, to spend a considerable part of each day with Jane the nurses would still need to have a great deal of information documented and readily available about the little girl's usual routines and independence in all the ALs in order to plan her nursing and, more important,

TABLE 3.1 JANE THOMSON: BACKGROUND NOTES TO ASSESSMENT OF ALs

AL	Guidelines to assessment
Maintaining a safe environment	Does the child engage in any particularly hazardous activities at present? (e.g., trying to climb out of cot)
	Does the child have any appreciation of danger? (e.g., of stairs, fire, hot foods)
	Does the child respond immediately to commands such as 'Stop!' 'No!'
Communicating	What words does the child speak?
	What other noises/vocalisations does the child use to refer to specific things/people?
	What gestures does the child use to communicate specific messages?
	How complex are the messages/instructions the child understands/responds to?
	How does the child communicate pleasure/anger/anxiety?
	Has the child ever been in hospital before?/had experience of doctors and nurses? (e.g., at clinic)
Breathing	Find our whether the child has ever had any problem affecting breathing and, if so, details.
	Observe/count breathing; count pulse; measure BP

minimise disruption to her particular routines. Enough is known about the possible harmful effects of hospitalisation on a child, that nowadays great care is taken to make sure that alteration of normal daily routines is minimal. Jane is at the age of being fairly independent in some ALs (e.g., eating and drinking) but still highly dependent in others (e.g., communicating). In addition, spending the major proportion of her time with her immediate family and in her home environment, she is likely still (unlike an older child at nursery) to have very rigid routines and have little experience of circumstances which demand alteration of these. The more familiar to her the nurses can make her day, the less frightened and anxious she should be.

Basic information about ALs likely to need attention overnight would be obtained from Mr Thomson before he returned home. The full assessment of ALs could be completed the next day with the help of Mrs Thomson and on the basis of the nurses' own observations of Jane.

The main purpose of this presentation is to illustrate how guidelines concerning assessing ALs given in the Introduction (pp. 1–4) are adapted in the case of the patient being a child. There follows, in note form for each AL, guidelines for assessing the young patient. Obviously the nurse would be guided in the assessment by her knowledge of child development and so notes are given of the level of dependence/independence in each AL which could be expected of a child of Jane's age. Finally, there are notes of the data obtained in the assessment of Jane's activities of living. These notes on each AL are, of course, only for explanation to readers. Only a summary of the data collected about the patient's ALs would be documented in the nursing notes. To illustrate this, a summary of these notes is provided on the right-hand side of Jane's Patient Assessment Form (Fig. 3.2, p. 28).

Indication of ability and dependence/independence at age 21 months	*Data collected about Jane*
Basically dependent on others for maintaining a safe environment. Has little concept of 'danger' but, through parental conditioning will have learned to avoid certain hazards, such as the fire, and responds to commands such as 'don't touch!' Because mobilising ability is now well developed and the child is impulsive, curious and adventurous, play is likely to involve dangers (e.g., from jumping off steps or objects, running, imitating adult activities such as using scissors).	Mother says that, despite the accident, Jane usually knows not to touch hot things. However, she admits that the child needs constant supervision to prevent accidents in the home. At present, most accidents—or their possibility—arise from Jane's interest in imitating her mother (e.g., getting up to the sink to wash dishes, standing on chairs to dust). Mother says Jane always responds to 'Stop that!' and 'Come here!' and 'No!'
By 21 months, the average child has begun to communicate verbally using understandable words—familiar words such as Mummy, Daddy, baby, bye bye. In addition, he may be able to repeat things said and join two words in speech (e.g., Daddy, bye bye). Various kinds of vocalisations and gestures enable the child to communicate effectively and to attract attention. The child of this age will enjoy scribbling, listening to music, being sung to and being shown and read picture books. He will not understand the meaning of time (e.g., 'Mummy is coming back tomorrow.') or explanation of unfamiliar things (e.g., 'The doctor is coming to see you.'). He may be able to answer 'yes/no questions' (e.g., 'Do you want juice?') but not questions such as 'What do you want to drink?' Crying outbursts and temper displays may be the child's only way of communicating discontent or frustration or fear. He will best understand reassurance if communicated non-verbally (by cuddling, rocking, stroking).	Mother says Jane 'chatters all the time', and can say Mummy, Daddy, baby, bed, juice, no, kisses, 'Letty' (name of lamb, her bedtime toy), potty, dolly. She can point to quite a few objects in books, if asked (e.g., banana, cake, duck, bus). She calls her grandmother 'na-na'. To get attention she cries or shouts 'Mummy' or if in the cot, rattles the cotsides. She shakes her head to communicate 'no' and nods to say 'yes'. She understands communications such as 'It's teatime/bedtime.' and responds to simple instructions such as 'Bring a nappy for the baby.', 'Get your potty.', 'Give Mummy a kiss.'. Jane's mother says she cries quite a lot when upset or wanting attention, especially if the baby is being attended to but, when happy, is affectionate and smiling.
Rate of respiration is about 25–35/minute in children age 2 Pulse rate: range of normal at age 2 is 80–140/minute Blood pressure: 80–90/60 at age 2	In outlining past medical history, Father had said Jane has often had colds. Does not have a cold at present, but nurses have observed that she has mucoid discharge from her nose which mother says is always there. Jane cannot wipe her nose herself.

TABLE 3.1 Continued

AL	Guidelines to assessment
Eating and drinking	What does the child usually eat and drink each day?
	Has he/she a good appetite?
	What foods/kind of food does he/she like best?
	Any particular dislikes?
	What does he/she prefer to drink?
	Can he/she feed himself/herself?
	What utensils does he/she use?
	Does he/she sit at table or in a highchair?
Eliminating	Does the child wear a nappy during day/night?
	If able to use potty/W.C. how does child indicate need to go?
	What words does he/she use for urine/faeces?
	How often/when does child open bowels?
Personal cleansing and dressing	What is the child's normal bathing/washing/hair washing routine?
	How much is the child able to manage without help?
	Does the child clean own teeth?/when?
	What is the state of the child's skin/hair/nails/teeth?
	How does the child normally dress?
	How independent in dressing is the child?
Controlling body temperature	Does the child show any signs of having an abnormally high/low temperature?
	Is the child's body temperature within the range of normal?
Mobilising	What stage of development in mobilising has the child reached?
	Does the child have any limitation on range of movement? If so, what?

Indication of ability and dependence/independence at age 21 months	*Data collected about Jane*
Balanced diet important, throughout childhood, for growth and prevention of obesity. Growth in second year slower than the tremendous increase in weight and size of first year of life. By age 2, average child is 90 cm (3 ft) tall and 15 kg (27 lb) in weight. By 21 months likely to be able to feed self without too much mess with spoon and fork (food cut up) sitting in a highchair. Will be able to drink from a 'feeder', perhaps from a cup. May be faddy about food at this age.	Jane's mother described her as a 'good eater' and able to feed herself (spoon only) quite well, although with much mess still. She has a cup of orange juice on waking at 0630 hours, then cereal with milk for breakfast; juice and a biscuit at 10; lunch at 12 midday: usually sausage and mash or fish fingers and beans, followed by custard or a banana; tea at 1700 hours: bread and jam and biscuits; warm milk before bed at 1900 hours. She prefers juice (orange) to milk; does not drink tea. She likes all sweet foods; dislikes vegetables (except potato and tinned beans). Especially likes ice cream, jelly, bread and jam. Jane has been reluctant to take drinks of juice overnight and this morning.
Development of control over elimination takes place between roughly 1½–3 years of age. Control of defaecation is achieved before control over micturition. Daytime continence precedes night-time continence.	Jane is still in nappies during day and night, but passes urine in potty if sat on it straight after meals. Does not indicate need to eliminate or having done so. She calls urine and faeces 'pee'. Usually has 1 or 2 bowel movements/day, always after breakfast and sometimes at teatime. Tends to have loose stools from time to time. Nurse observed that nappy removed in the morning was strong smelling and slightly discoloured.
Toddlers usually like bathtime and enjoy learning to gain independence in personal cleansing and dressing activities. At 21 months a child may be able to partially wash using soap and sponge in the bath, but will need help to finish and to be dried. Dependent for care of finger and toe nails. Should be able to attempt to brush and comb hair, but will need help. Perhaps able to attempt to brush teeth but will need assistance to brush all thoroughly and must be prompted to carry out this activity. The milk teeth grow in between 6 months and 6 years; teething is often painful, even to a toddler; prevention of dental caries is important. By 21 months the child will begin to recognise (and bring, if asked) garments of clothing and may attempt to dress, e.g., put on socks.	Being without a fixed bath or hot water supply, Jane is used to a twice weekly all over wash in the kitchen sink and a weekly hair wash. Her mother confessed that Jane does not have a toothbrush and has never been taught to brush her teeth. The nurse observed that Jane's nails are ragged and dirty and her overall standard of cleanliness is poor. Her hair is short and looks clean. Jane is accustomed to wearing dungarees with a jumper and socks underneath. She is beginning to help to dress herself.

Average body temperature at 2 years: 37.8°C
 	
A young child's temperature can change more quickly and dramatically than an adult's because thermoregulation is less efficient. Raised temperature does not necessarily result in raised pulse rate in young child.
	Temperature recorded:
	  at 2200 hours Saturday 38.2°C
	  at 0600 hours Sunday 37.8°C
	  at 1000 hours Sunday 38.0°C
	
	Jane observed to be flushed and skin rather hot and dry on waking on Sunday.

Independent mobilising is one of the most important and obvious acquisitions of the first 2 years, progressing through raising head, sitting, crawling, standing, walking, managing stairs, jumping, running, hopping and skipping. Agility and speed increase with practice. Between about 18 months and 2 years stairs, jumping and running are mastered.	Jane is described by her parents as an active little girl. She has recently learned to walk downstairs, holding the rail, without help. She tends to trip and fall when running about.

TABLE 3.1 Continued

AL	*Guidelines to assessment*
Working and playing	What toys/type of toy does the child most enjoy?
	Does the child have a particular toy to take to bed?
	What kind of toy/play is likely to be most enjoyed during time in hospital?
Expressing sexuality	In what ways does the child portray femininity/masculinity?
	Might the current health problem/hospitalisation affect sexual development?
Sleeping	What is the child's usual bedtime/time of waking?
	Does the child waken during the night? If so, when? and why?

	Does the child sleep in a bed/cot?
	    with/without a pillow?
	    with others in the room?
	    with light on/off?
	    with favourite toy?
	    in heated/unheated room?
	    with blankets/duvet?

	Does the child have a daytime sleep? If so, when?
	Does the child seem to be having sufficient rest and sleep?

Indication of ability and dependence/independence at age 21 months	*Data collected about Jane*
Play occupies much of a toddler's time: games, such as brick building, scribbling and ball; imitative play, such as washing dishes, using tea set; and imaginative play with dolls and soft toys. Books now capture more sustained attention and the child can turn pages one or two at a time.	Jane's mother was able to list several favourite toys—her 'playpeople', nursery rhyme books, dolls, a saucepan set—and said she had brought in Jane's lamb (called 'Letty') which Jane took to bed and liked to cuddle and suck whenever tired or miserable. Jane was used to amusing herself because her mother was busy with the baby. She was beginning to enjoy television, especially cartoons.
Young children enjoy being cuddled, rocked and stroked because human beings have an innate sensuality. The toddler, especially once toilet trained, may show interest in his/her genital area and may embarrass parents by using so-called 'rude words' in public. At this age, modesty is not developed and the toddler is unlikely to have any concern at being exposed or handled by nurses and doctors.	No specific questions were put to Jane's parents about this AL but, in the course of discussion, several references were made to the fact that part of Jane's neck and chest had been scalded. Obviously her parents were anxious that there may be permanent disfigurement as a result of the burns.
Sleep is essential for growth and sleeping is a predominant activity in childhood. The average number of hours spent sleeping by a child of 21 months would be between 12–14 hours. This may consist of 10–12 hours at night (e.g., 7 pm–7 am) and a nap (1–2 hours) morning or afternoon. Toddlers may resist going to bed and may be disturbed by dreams or nightmares. Routine is important, especially a routine schedule and quietening activities (e.g., reading) before bedtime.	Jane is described by her parents as a 'bad sleeper'. She tends to become 'difficult' (crying, aggressive) when bedtime is announced, cries when put in her cot and often wakes and cries early in the morning (4 am approximately). Sometimes this bedtime protest is ignored and she is allowed to stay up till she falls asleep, or else she is left to cry in cot. Bedtime is between 5 and 9 pm; she is usually taken into the parents' bed about 6.30 am. She sleeps for 1 to 1½ hours after lunch. Jane sleeps in a cot, without a pillow, with 2 blankets (she wears a sleeping suit) and her toy lamb. Her cot is in the parents bedroom (the whole family share one room). The room is unheated and the light is put off when the parents go to sleep.

Patient Assessment Form

Date of admission	*4 March*	Date of assessment	*4 March*

Surname   *STEVENSON*   Forenames   *Harold*

Male	✓	Age	79	~~Single~~/~~Married~~/*Recently* Widowed	Prefers to be addressed as
Female				Other	*Mr Stevenson*

Date of birth

Address of usual residence   *Millstone Cottage*
Costertown
near Newtown

Type of accommodation   *One storey, 3 roomed cottage. Modernised. Small bathroom, indoor toil*
hot water supply. Coal fire.

Family/Others at this residence   *None*

Next of kin   Name *James Stevenson*   Address *215 Pickering Park Avenue*
Redwood

Relationship *Eldest son*   Tel. no. *South Australia 5077*

Significant others   Relatives/Dependents *Eldest son (see above), married, 3 married children with*
2 children each. Other son lives 150 miles away✱; married w
2 children

✱ address to contact:
2 Main Street   Helpers ⎫
Altonville.   ⎬ *Neighbours*
Tel: Altonville 716   Visitors ⎭

Occupation   *Retired bricklayer*

Religious beliefs and relevant practices   *Devout Methodist. Attends village chapel when taken by car.*

Patient's perception of current health status   *Feels unwell, unable to get over wife's recent death.*
Knows he has 'a heart condition'.

Reason for ~~admission~~/referral *(to H.V.)*   *Frailty, recently bereaved.*

Medical diagnosis   *Mild chronic congestive cardiac failure.*

Past medical history   *CCF for 10 years. Treated for anaemia (iron deficiency) 5 years ago.*
Hospitalised with pneumonia when aged 60.

Allergies   *None*   Significant life crises   *Wife died in February this y*
(golden wedding anniversar
celebrated in March last yr.

Fig 3.3 Mr Stevenson: first assessment of ALs

Assessment of Activities of Living ① Date *4 March*

Patient's problems
(actual/potential)
(p) = potential

AL	Usual routines: what he/she can and cannot do independently
● Maintaining a safe environment	House tidy; floors trip-free; no trailing flexes. Kitchenette clean. Says he is very careful about the open coal fire; uses a fire guard.
● Communicating	Pleasant manner; reasonable vocabulary. Only slightly hard of hearing. Sight good. Apparent sorrow when talking of the loss of his wife.
● Breathing	No recent respiratory infection; no cough; no cyanosis or breathlessness. Has never smoked.
● Eating and drinking	Had never cooked until wife's death. Has bread and marmalade for breakfast; soup and a sandwich for lunch; bread and jam and cake for tea; cocoa and biscuit at 2100 hrs. Has full dentures.
● Eliminating	Passes urine x 6 daily and x 1 during night; slight urgency, no incontinence. Has always been constipated; takes 2 Beecham's pills every other night.
● Personal cleansing and dressing	Used to bath weekly but has not used bath since wife died for fear of slipping. Washes morning and evening; soaks dentures overnight; a neighbour cuts his hair and does his personal washing each week.
● Controlling body temperature	Kitchen feels warm, but his hands are cold. Puts an electric fire on in bedroom for an hour at bedtime. Knows of danger of hypothermia.
● Mobilising	Easily tired. Has not been out much in last month; would like to feel well enough to go out for walks.
● Working and playing	Retired bricklaying at 70. Now listens to the radio, watches TV selectively, reads spy stories. Since retiring has shared all his time with his wife.
● Expressing sexuality	Nil of relevance.
● Sleeping	Previously a good sleeper; disturbed over last month. Does not believe in taking sleeping pills. Does not worry about being awake.
● Dying	

MR HAROLD STEVENSON   Age 79

Old and alone

The district nurses and the health visitors worked from the health centre in the city, five miles away from the small village in which old Mr Stevenson lived. His doctor was in the habit of visiting Mr Stevenson monthly to check on his chronic heart condition. At his most recent visit he was shocked to see how frail and unresponsive Mr Stevenson had become in the short time since the death of Mrs Stevenson.

At the next staff conference it was decided that Mr Stevenson should be assessed on a regular basis for a while by one of the health visitors so that, if necessary, support services could become involved in the care of this elderly man.

FIRST ASSESSMENT

The health visitor assigned to Mr Stevenson was able to prepare for her first assessment interview by recording on the Patient Assessment Form (Fig. 3.3) some of the biographical and health data already available. She also had a personal discussion with the district nurses who had looked after Mrs Stevenson at home during her recent short terminal illness which followed a very severe stroke. This helped the health visitor to prepare herself psychologically for meeting this elderly, recently bereaved man.

After locating his cottage, she rang the doorbell and noticed that Mr Stevenson took some time to answer and open the door. However, he seemed pleased to see the health visitor and to be addressed by name, even at her first visit. She was invited into the living room where, she noticed, a small coal fire was burning. She wondered whether or not this presented a fire risk.

The health visitor realised that before starting her assessment, they both needed to acknowledge and talk about Mr Stevenson's recent bereavement. As their initial conversation had not been difficult the health visitor decided she could broach the subject. Of course there were tears but once they abated Mr Stevenson was eager to talk about his wife and family. He said that with both his sons so far away he felt very alone now, although not too lonely. The younger son phoned twice a week and he and his wife visited every two months or so. The elder son wrote every week and sent photographs regularly. They all understood that Mr Stevenson wanted to continue living in the cottage which had been his home for so long.

This was an appropriate cue for the health visitor to find out what he could and could not do in relation to his ALs.

Mr Stevenson seemed to enjoy talking about himself and his daily living activities. Despite being widowed so recently, Mr Stevenson appeared to be making a determined effort to cope independently at home.

The data collected in this first assessment are summarised in Figure 3.3 on page 36.

SECOND ASSESSMENT

One month later, in April, the health visitor returned to see Mr Stevenson and a second assessment of his ALs was carried out. The data collected on this occasion are presented in Figure 3.4. By comparing Figure 3.4 with 3.3 readers will be able to ascertain the changes which occurred in the month between the first and second assessments.

THIRD ASSESSMENT

In May a further assessment was made by the health visitor. Data collected are presented in Figure 3.5 and, if readers compare this with data obtained in the two previous assessments (Figs. 3.4 and 3.3) further improvement will be evident.

For those nurses who in their work only make periodic visits to their patients, collection of data in a systematic way about the ALs gives an overall estimation of what patients can manage to do themselves and what is becoming difficult or impossible. Such intermittent assessment is invaluable in monitoring increasing, decreasing or unchanged ability in relation to each AL. In Mr Stevenson's case it is to be expected, because of his age and chronic heart condition, that he will become increasingly less independent in carrying out his ALs.

However, the objective in collecting assessment data is to identify the patient's problems, both actual and potential. The sooner problems are identified, the sooner intervention to solve, alleviate or prevent the problems can be implemented. In the next chapter the procedure of *identifying patients' problems* is discussed and illustrated.

REFERENCE

Kratz C (ed) 1979 The nursing process. Balliere Tindall, London, p 21

Assessment of Activities of Living ② Date 4 April

Mr Harold STEVENSON

AL	Usual routines: what he/she can and cannot do independently
● Maintaining a safe environment	House remains safe. Still dealing safely with open fire.
● Communicating	No change, except that he seems more relaxed and cheerful. Talked openly about his wife with less distress than before.
● Breathing	No change.
● Eating and drinking	For 2 weeks has had lunch delivered by meals-on-wheels three times a week. Has eaten and enjoyed these. Is eating cheese or meat at teatime now and 'All Bran' for breakfast. Has gained weight
● Eliminating	Is delighted that changed diet has resulted in daily bowel movement (except one day) Has stopped taking aperients.
● Personal cleansing and dressing	Has now a slip-mat in the bath but is awaiting grab rails. Did not accept offer of bath attendant.
● Controlling body temperature	Hands cold as before but room temperature seems adequate and warm clothing being worn.
● Mobilising	Less easily fatigued. Has been out for a short walk on several days. Was taken by car to chapel last Sunday.
● Working and playing	Knowledgeable about recent radio and TV programmes.
● Expressing sexuality	
● Sleeping	Often unable to get to sleep; wakes early (0500 hrs). However, does not feel tired.
● Dying	

Fig. 3.4 Mr Stevenson: second assessment of ALs

Assessment of Activities of Living ③

Mr Harold STEVENSON

Date *12 May*

Patient's problems
(actual/potential)
(p) = potential

AL	Usual routines: what he/she can and cannot do independently
● Maintaining a safe environment	No evidence of deterioration in safety standards
● Communicating	Continues to be more cheerful.
● Breathing	Is experiencing shortness of breath at times (eg. carrying in coal).
● Eating and drinking	Continues to appreciate Meals-on-Wheels and to eat a more varied diet, including dietary fibre. Has gained additional weight; looks much stronger.
● Eliminating	Daily bowel movement / no constipation if 'All Bran' taken daily.
● Personal cleansing and dressing	Grab rails now fixed in bathroom. Has had 2 baths and feels confident about bathing alone.
● Controlling body temperature	Hands not so cold. Weather now warmer; house sufficiently warm.
● Mobilising	Has walked to the village shop each day, except when raining. Feels more energetic / less tired after activity.
● Working and playing	No evidence of boredom or depression. Seems to fill the days to his satisfaction.
● Expressing sexuality	
● Sleeping	Is sleeping better and feels more refreshed on waking.
● Dying	

Fig. 3.5 Mr Stevenson : third assessment of ALs

4

Identifying patients' problems

Having collected data about the patient's ALs from assessment, the next step in the process of nursing is to inspect those data and identify the patient's problems.

For example, if a patient had described to the nurse that whenever he ate fried foods he developed indigestion and felt sick, she could state his problem as:

- indigestion/nausea due to fried foods

This is an *actual problem*: i.e., it actually exists at present. A second category of problem is described as a *potential problem* (abbreviated as (p) on the Patient Assessment Form). This type is identified on the basis of data collected which suggests that the patient might, in the future, develop a problem. To take an obvious example, if a patient is very thin, confined to bed, occasionally incontinent and sometimes confused, then it can be predicted that this patient is:

- at risk of developing pressure sores

This is a *potential* problem.

That last example is also interesting in that the patient himself may not perceive that this potential problem exists. Thus a distinction can be made between 'patient-perceived' and 'nurse-perceived' problems. Another example of a problem which might be perceived by the nurse but not by the patient is that, on the basis of his description of his usual drinking habits, he appears to be:

- dependent upon alcohol

It is quite possible that this patient, far from considering his habits a problem, views drinking as a pleasurable activity. However, if the nurse discussed with him her concern, the patient may come to realise that he does have a problem and may request help or be willing to be helped.

In fact, confirming with the patient the existence of problems identified by the nurse from assessment data is a necessary activity. It is important that both the nurse and patient agree that those identified problems are, indeed, problems.

Once this is agreed, the problems identified are written unambiguously on the Patient Assessment Form. The data

on which identification of these problems was made should be clearly stated. As data from subsequent assessment and evaluation show that problems have been solved, or are not being solved, or that new ones have developed, the problem list is updated accordingly.

The three patients introduced in Chapter 3 are re-introduced now to illustrate the procedure of problem identification. Their Patient Assessment Forms are now complete, including a list of the problems identified on the basis of the assessment data, in relation to the ALs.

MR MITCHELL'S PROBLEMS

Analysis of Mr Mitchell's assessment data as displayed in Figure 3.1 (p. 26) reveals that he had problems other than haematuria, the reason for admission. Worry and anxiety is his other main problem. Top of the list of causes of his anxiety is the speed with which he was admitted to hospital after visiting his doctor. There is so much publicity about long waiting lists, it is understandable that an almost immediate summons to hospital suggests to a lay person the possible gravity of the condition. This can make a person feel very threatened.

The next cause of anxiety was the reason for his admission—cystoscopy and biopsy to investigate the cause of his haematuria. Another possible cause was the recent separation from his wife, since he said that she was not to be contacted without his permission.

Looking again at the assessment data there is also a *potential problem*—the health risks associated with smoking. These identified problems are set out below and also stated on the completed Patient Assessment Form (Fig. 4.1):

Patient Assessment Form

Date of admission   *6 May*

Date of assessment   *6 May*

Surname   *MITCHELL*

Forenames   *Gordon Peter*

Male   [✓]
Female   [ ]

Age   *48*

Date of birth

Single / Married✓ / Widowed

Other   *but separated from wife*

Prefers to be addressed as

Mr Mitchell

Address of usual residence   *13 High Street, Newtown*

Type of accommodation   *Flat above business premises*

Family/Others at this residence   *Lives alone*

Next of kin ✱   Name   *Anne Mitchell*

Address   *4 Hillview Crescent Newtown*

Relationship   *Wife (separated)*

Tel. no.   ————

✱ Not inform of admission to be contacte without patic permissio

Significant others   Relatives/Dependents   *2 adult sons (neither informed of admission)*

Helpers   ————

Visitors   *No family visitors. Partner (J. Davey) may visit.*

Occupation   *Architect: own business with one partner*

Religious beliefs and relevant practices   *Roman Catholic*

Patient's perception of current health status   *Understands that haematuria indicates some dysfunction of the urinary system and requires investigation*

Reason for admission/referral   *Investigation of haematuria: cystoscopy and biopsy*

Medical diagnosis   *None, as yet*

Past medical history   *Appendix removed at age 17.*

Allergies   *None*

Significant life crises   *Recently separated from wife*

Fig. 4.1 Mr Mitchell: first assessment with problems stated

Assessment of Activities of Living

Date *6 May*

AL	Usual routines: what he/she can and cannot do independently	Patient's problems (actual/potential) (p) = potential
● Maintaining a safe environment	*Independent*	
● Communicating	*Fluent, articulate in speech. Communicates with ease. Conveys anxiety about forthcoming investigation / possible causes of haematuria.*	● *Worry / anxiety due to: speed of admission, reason for admission, significant life crisis*
● Breathing	*Smokes 15 cigarettes per day. Has a productive morning cough. Does not become breathless on exertion.*	● *(p) Health risks from smoking*
● Eating and drinking	*Good appetite. Is not overweight. Prefers natural foodstuffs. Dislikes fish and eggs. Does not drink alcohol in excess.*	
● Eliminating	*Apart from recent onset of haematuria and dysuria, micturition is normal. Bowels regular (daily)*	● *Haematuria*
● Personal cleansing and dressing	*Meticulous standard of cleanliness and grooming. Showers and shaves daily (am). Wears full dentures.*	
● Controlling body temperature	*Body temperature within range of normal on admission.*	
● Mobilising	*Full range of movement. Very active. Jogs daily. Swims regularly.*	
● Working and playing	*Business (architecture) is main activity and interest in life, especially since recent separation from wife. Plays squash weekly.*	
● Expressing sexuality	*Nil of note*	
● Sleeping	*Good sleeper; retires at 2330 hrs, rises at 0600 hrs. Does not take sleeping tablets.*	
● Dying		

actual problems {
- worry and anxiety caused by
  speed of admission
  reason for admission
  significant recent life crisis
- haematuria

potential problems {
- health risks from smoking

These then are Mr Mitchell's problems identified by the nurse from the data. The next step in the procedure is discussion with Mr Mitchell as to whether or not he perceives these as problems. He admitted his anxiety and talked freely about it and even mentioned cancer of the bladder as a possibility. He also talked about his personal worries thus confirming them as contributory factors to his overall anxiety level. When the subject of smoking was introduced he was well aware of the risks to health but was willing to take the risk. This does not stop his smoking being a potential problem, it only means that he is not prepared to take action to prevent this potential problem from becoming an actual one.

JANE THOMSON'S PROBLEMS

From Jane's assessment data (Fig. 3.2, p. 28) it is obvious that within a very short time this 21-month-old girl had suddenly been presented with a considerable number of problems, the immediate ones being:
- soreness and pain from the scalds
- limitation of movement due to splinted arm
- separation from her parents and home

Any discontinuity of the skin renders a person vulnerable to infection and in Jane's case there was considerable skin loss so that an additional potential problem was:
- infected skin

On waking the next morning Jane had two additional problems, firstly she was flushed and hot, and an increased body temperature was confirmed objectively by a clinical thermometer. Secondly she faced disruption of her normal daily routine which is very disturbing to a child of this age. These additional problems can be stated as:
- increased body temperature
- disruption of daily routine

When Jane's mother arrived she helped the nurse to complete the assessment data and from this additional information, the nurse identified several more problems:
- 'runny' nose
- lack of dental hygiene
- overcrowded/hazardous home environment

And any person after a scald has a potential problem:
- disfigurement

These various problems are listed on Jane's Patient Assessment Form (Fig. 4.2, p. 46) alongside the relevant ALs.

MR STEVENSON'S PROBLEMS

Mr Stevenson was initially referred to the health visiting list because his doctor was concerned about deterioration in his condition following the death of his wife. Data from the health visitor's *first assessment* (Fig. 3.3) confirmed the existence of these two problems:
- frailty
- grieving

But it also revealed several other problems, verified by Mr Stevenson as problematic. The prime one was his inadequate diet because of his inability to cook and his lack of knowledge. As he looked malnourished, the problem was stated as:
- malnutrition

He volunteered that he had 'always been constipated' and regularly took laxative pills, two every other night. These problems were identified as:
- constipation
- over-reliance on aperients

Data from the first assessment revealed that he was easily fatigued and had not felt inclined to go out since his wife's death. The problems were identified as:
- inadequate exercise
- lack of fresh air

The data also stated that he had not bathed since his wife's death because he was afraid of slipping when in the house alone. The problem was identified as:
- loss of confidence for bathing

Because of his frailty and the open fire the health visitor identified a potential problem:
- fire risk

And although the kitchen felt sufficiently warm, when the health visitor shook Mr Stevenson's hand in greeting, it was very cold. These data permitted identification of another potential problem:
- hypothermia

Without assessment of Mr Stevenson's ALs it is likely that these problems would not have been identified. Identifying them is the first step towards helping a patient to deal with them. The problems identified above (both actual and potential) are stated on Mr Stevenson's Patient Assessment Form (Fig. 4.3, p. 48) alongside the relevant ALs.

In Figure 4.4 (p. 50) Mr Stevenson's problems identified after the *second assessment* are listed as:

- grieving
- unwilling to use bath (awaiting grab rails)
- difficulty in sleeping/waking early

In Figure 4.5 (p. 51) Mr Stevenson's circumstances at the *third assessment* are described and, at this time, there is only one major health problem apparent:

- slight breathlessness on exertion

Patient Assessment Form

| Date of admission | *10 November* | | Date of assessment | *10 November* |

Surname　*THOMSON*　　　　　Forenames *Jane*

Male ☐
Female ☑

Age / Date of birth　*21/12*

Single/Married/Widowed
Other

Prefers to be addressed as
Jane

Address of usual residence　*213 Bridge Road, Billington*

Type of accommodation　*Small flat; shared w.c.; no bath/hot water supply*

Family/~~Others~~ at this residence　*Parents and baby brother*

Next of kin　Name　*John Thomson*　　　Address　*as above*
　　　　　　Relationship　*Father*　　　Tel. no. *{of neighbour (Mrs Brown) 022-73231*
　　　　　　　　　　　　　　　　　　　　　　　{of grandmother's work (am) 022-847...

Significant others　Relatives/~~Dependents~~　*Parents. Baby brother (4 months) - Michael*

　　　　　　　　　Helpers

　　　　　　　　　Visitors　*Maternal grandparents*

Occupation　*(Father's) Unemployed factory worker*

Religious beliefs and relevant practices　*No religion*

Patient's perception of current health status

Reason for admission/~~referral~~　*Burns from scalding accident at home.*

Medical diagnosis　*Superficial burns: part neck, chest, R arm*

Past medical history　*Frequent colds. No serious illness / no previous hospital admission*

Allergies　*None*　　　　　　　　　　Significant life crises

Fig. 4.2 Jane Thomson: first assessment with problems stated

Assessment of Activities of Living

Date *10/11 Nov*

Patient's problems
(actual/potential)
(p) = potential

AL	Usual routines: what he/she can and cannot do independently	
● Maintaining a safe environment	Dependent on others for safety. Does respond to 'No!' and 'Stop that!' Currently prone to accidents/falls when imitating adults' activities.	● Overcrowded/hazardous home environment
● Communicating	Has started to speak; single words (Mummy, Daddy, baby, bed, juice, no, kisses, "Letty"= Lamb, potty). Understands/responds to simple phrases.	
● Breathing	Constantly runny nose; frequent colds. Respirations 35/minute on admission; pulse 128/min	● Runny nose
● Eating and drinking	'Good eater'; able to spoonfeed self. Juice at 0630; breakfast-cereal; lunch at 1200, eg sausages); tea at 1700; milk before bed; prefers juice to milk/sweet foods to savoury. Reluctant to drink since admission	
● Eliminating	In nappies at all times. Uses potty after meals. B.O. after breakfast/tea. Stools sometimes loose. Refers to stools and urine as "pee." Strong-smelling nappy this a.m.	
● Personal cleansing and dressing	Used to twice weekly 'bath' in sink/weekly hairwash. Observed to have dirty, ragged nails. Does not clean teeth. Likes to help wash/dress self.	● Soreness from scalds ● (p) Infected skin ● Lack of dental hygiene
● Controlling body temperature	Temperature at 2200 hrs Saturday (10/10) 38.2°C 0600 hrs Sunday (11/10) 37.8°C 1000 hrs Sunday (11/10) 38.0°C Flushed and hot on waking this am.	● Increased body temperature
● Mobilising	Active child. Full range of movement. Has recently learned to walk downstairs, holding rail.	● Limitation of movement due to splinted arm
● Working and playing	Plays well by self. Favourite toys: 'play people', books, dolls, saucepan set, toy lamb ("Letty"). Loves being read to (especially nursery rhymes).	● Separation from parents and home ● Disruption of daily routine
● Expressing sexuality	Parents anxious about possibility of permanent disfigurement from burns.	● (p) Disfigurement
● Sleeping	'Bad sleeper.' Cries at bedtime (1700-2100 hrs); wakes crying, approx 0400. Wakens about 0630. Sleeps in cot in room with rest of family. No pillow; sleepsuit and 2 blankets.	
● Dying		

Patient Assessment Form

Date of admission	*4 March*
Date of assessment	*4 March*

Surname *STEVENSON*   Forenames *Harold*

Male [✓]   Age **79**   ~~Single~~/~~Married~~/Widowed *Recently*   Prefers to be addressed as

Female [ ]   Date of birth   Other   *Mr Stevenson*

Address of usual residence *Millstone Cottage, Costertown, near Newtown*

Type of accommodation *One storey, 3 roomed cottage. Modernised. Small bathroom, indoor toilet, hot water supply. Coal fire.*

Family/Others at this residence *None*

Next of kin   Name *James Stevenson*   Address *215 Pickering Park Avenue Redwood*

Relationship *Eldest son*   Tel. no. *South Australia 5077*

Significant others   Relatives/Dependents *Eldest son (see above), married, 3 married children with 2 children each. Other son lives 150 miles away * married with 2 children.*

＊ address to contact: 2 Main Street Altonville. Tel: Altonville 716   Helpers } *Neighbours*   Visitors

Occupation *Retired bricklayer*

Religious beliefs and relevant practices *Devout Methodist. Attends village chapel when taken by car.*

Patient's perception of current health status *Feels unwell, unable to get over wife's recent death. Knows he has 'a heart condition'.*

Reason for ~~admission~~/referral *(to H.V.) Frailty, recently bereaved.*

Medical diagnosis *Mild chronic congestive cardiac failure.*

Past medical history *CCF for 10 years. Treated for anaemia (iron deficiency) 5 years ago. Hospitalised with pneumonia when aged 60.*

Allergies *None.*   Significant life crises *Wife died in February this year (golden wedding anniversary celeb in March last year.)*

Fig. 4.3 Mr Stevenson: first assessment with problems stated

Assessment of Activities of Living   ① Date 4 March

AL	Usual routines: what he/she can and cannot do independently	Patient's problems (actual/potential) (p) = potential
● Maintaining a safe environment	House tidy; floors trip-free; no trailing flexes. Kitchenette clean. Says he is very careful about the open coal fire; uses a fire guard.	● (p) Fire risk
● Communicating	Pleasant manner; reasonable vocabulary. Only slightly hard of hearing. Sight good. Apparent sorrow when talking of the loss of his wife.	● Grieving
● Breathing	No recent respiratory infection; no cough; no cyanosis or breathlessness. Has never smoked.	● Lack of fresh air
● Eating and drinking	Had never cooked until wife's death. Has bread and marmalade for breakfast; soup and a sandwich for lunch; bread and jam and cake for tea; cocoa and biscuit at 2100 hrs. Has full dentures.	● Frailty ● Malnutrition
● Eliminating	Passes urine x 6 daily and x1 during night; slight urgency, no incontinence. Has always been constipated; takes 2 Beecham's pills every other night.	● Constipated ● Over-reliance on aperients
● Personal cleansing and dressing	Used to bath weekly, but has not used bath since wife died for fear of slipping. Washes morning and evening; soaks dentures overnight; a neighbour cuts his hair and does his personal washing each week.	● Loss of confidence for bathing
● Controlling body temperature	Kitchen feels warm, but his hands are cold. Puts an electric fire on in bedroom for an hour at bedtime. Knows of danger of hypothermia.	● (p) Hypothermia
● Mobilising	Easily tired. Has not been out much in last month; would like to feel well enough to go out for walks.	● Inadequate exercise
● Working and playing	Retired bricklaying at 70. Now listens to the radio, watches TV selectively, reads spy stories. Since retiring has shared all his time with his wife.	
● Expressing sexuality	Nil of relevance.	
● Sleeping	Previously a good sleeper; disturbed over last month. Does not believe in taking sleeping pills. Does not worry about being awake.	
● Dying		

Assessment of Activities of Living ②

Date *4 April*

Mr Harold STEVENSON

Patient's problems
(actual/potential)
(p) = potential

AL	Usual routines: what he/she can and cannot do independently	
● Maintaining a safe environment	*House remains safe. Still dealing safely with open fire.*	
● Communicating	*No change, except that he seems more relaxed and cheerful. Talked openly about his wife with less distress than before.*	● *Grieving*
● Breathing	*No change.*	
● Eating and drinking	*For 2 weeks has had lunch delivered by meals-on-wheels three times a week. Has eaten and enjoyed these. Is eating cheese or meat at teatime now and 'All Bran' for breakfast. Has gained weight.*	
● Eliminating	*Is delighted that changed diet has resulted in daily bowel movement (except one day). Has stopped taking aperients.*	
● Personal cleansing and dressing	*Has now a slip-mat in the bath but is awaiting grab rails. Did not accept offer of bath attendant.*	● *Unwilling to use bath*
● Controlling body temperature	*Hands cold as before but room temperature seems adequate and warm clothing being worn.*	
● Mobilising	*Less easily fatigued. Has been out for a short walk on several days. Was taken by car to chapel last Sunday.*	
● Working and playing	*Knowledgeable about recent radio and TV programmes.*	
● Expressing sexuality		
● Sleeping	*Often unable to get to sleep; wakes early (0500 hrs). However, does not feel tired.*	● *Difficulty in sleeping / waking early.*
● Dying		

Fig. 4.4 Mr Stevenson: second assessment with problems stated

Assessment of Activities of Living ③

Date *12 May*

Mr Harold STEVENSON

AL	Usual routines: what he/she can and cannot do independently	Patient's problems (actual/potential) (p) = potential
● Maintaining a safe environment	*No evidence of deterioration in safety standards.*	
● Communicating	*Continues to be more cheerful*	
● Breathing	*Is experiencing shortness of breath at times (eg. carrying in coal).*	● *Slight breathlessness on exertion*
● Eating and drinking	*Continues to appreciate meals-on-wheels and to eat a more varied diet, including dietary fibre. Has gained additional weight; looks much stronger.*	
● Eliminating	*Daily bowel movement / no constipation if 'All Bran' taken daily.*	
● Personal cleansing and dressing	*Grab rails now fixed in bathroom. Has had 2 baths and feels confident about bathing alone.*	
● Controlling body temperature	*Hands not so cold. Weather now warmer; house sufficiently warm.*	
● Mobilising	*Has walked to the village shop each day, except when raining. Feels more energetic / less tired after activity.*	
● Working and playing	*No evidence of boredom or depression. Seems to fill the days to his satisfaction.*	
● Expressing sexuality		
● Sleeping	*Is sleeping better and feels more refreshed on waking.*	
● Dying		

Fig. 4.5 Mr Stevenson: third assessment with problems stated

5

Identifying patients' learning needs

In the previous chapter, identifying patients' problems was the topic discussed and illustrated, but as the nurse also plays an important *teaching* role in contemporary health care, we shall now look at the subject of identifying patients' learning needs.

Health education and patient teaching have become more and more important as it has been realised that the 'self-care' concept is crucial to modern society and to the economic viability of a nation's health care system.

These activities are important in all branches of nursing and in every health care setting. The health education role of the health visitor, especially with young children and increasingly with the elderly, is probably widely recognised. Teaching patients to cope with a stoma (colostomy or ileostomy) is a function of hospital nurses, community nurses and sometimes, nurses specially trained as stoma therapists. As illustrated in Chapter 11 pre-operative teaching is fast coming to be regarded as an important job of nurses in surgical wards. Teaching as part of a patient's rehabilitation is illustrated, specifically in relation to a patient who has had a myocardial infarction, (Ch. 13, p. 101).

It is beginning to be realised in nursing that teaching is a complex and skilled activity and, like any other nursing intervention, it is likely to be more effectively implemented if it is carefully planned. Once again, the process of nursing provides an appropriate framework for considering teaching in nursing.

The following presentation illustrates the first step in the process of patient teaching—*identifying patients' learning needs*. The patient is Kate Warrender, an adolescent who is found to need re-education in relation to her diabetic condition.

KATE WARRENDER Age 17½

Problems with diabetes mellitus

Kate was well used to her diabetic condition as the diagnosis had been made when she was eight years old. The condition had been well controlled and she said she had not really felt handicapped by it. But since she left school 18 months ago, she had had four admissions to hospital, this one being the fifth.

However, during the current admission careful probing revealed that Kate (and her family) did not really understand some aspects of the control of Kate's diabetes at the present time. Therefore, the focus of this study is the identification, from data collected at an assessment interview, of Kate's learning needs.

Kate had had a sore toe for a few days and when it started to throb she went to her doctor's morning surgery and he prescribed a course of oral antibiotics. Later in the evening she felt unwell, irritable and tired. Her urine showed 2 per cent glucose so she increased the dose of insulin. The next morning there was still 2 per cent glucose in her urine and ketones + +; she had epigastric pain and polyuria and felt nauseated, anorexic, dyspnoeic, dehydrated and thirsty—all the classical signs and symptoms of diabetic ketoacidosis. By the time that she was admitted to the ward at 1100 hours she felt ill and miserable. Skilled medical and nursing treatment throughout the day achieved its objective; her urine in the late evening contained 0.5 per cent glucose and by the next morning it was glucose-free. So on the second day Kate was feeling much better and was happy to discuss with the nurse the problems she had been having in controlling her diabetes.

Basic biographical and health data are contained in the left-hand side of Kate's Patient Assessment Form (Fig.

5.1). Data about ALs are on the right-hand side of that form.

Kate was an attractive girl who obviously enjoyed being well groomed and dressed. She had a pleasant manner, a nice smile and seemed to enjoy talking about herself and her family. Her older brother was 20 and in the police force; her younger brother was 16 and would be leaving school in the summer—he wanted to join the army. Her younger sister of 12 was doing well at school—she was the 'brainy' one of the family. Kate shared a bedroom with her sister. Her mother now worked full-time as a manageress of a small shop; her father was a factory foreman, working shifts to earn more money.

Kate felt that her father had always been less interested in and worried about her diabetic condition than her mother. Although Kate said that she looked after her diet, urine testing and injections, she said that it was her mother who noticed when the condition seemed to be going out of balance and warned Kate. In fact, Kate had thought recently that her mother was too protective towards her and, now that she was older, she was beginning to resent this. Asked about her attitude towards being diabetic, Kate said she did not really feel handicapped by her condition. However, further probing revealed that it did make a difference in the family. Kate considered that, although the second oldest child, she was treated as much younger and was beginning to be irritated about this. Kate agreed that one of her present needs was:

• to reconsider, in the light of growing up, what 'being diabetic' means

In adulthood, having diabetes essentially means accepting total responsibility oneself for adhering to a strict routine, being alert to signals of imbalance and carrying out the lifelong treatment regime day in, day out—not with the objective of pleasing parents or impressing friends, but solely to enable the body to function within physiological norms.

Kate also volunteered the information that she was worried about the future; she knew a little about the possible complications of diabetes, but was unsure how these could affect her. Just recently she had an added anxiety because her menstrual cycle had become very irregular: her last period was three months ago. Her anxiety about diabetes 'being passed on' arose quite naturally when she talked about going to the pub and to the cinema with her boyfriend; she wondered if a boy might have reservations about marrying a diabetic. Asked if she would like to have children she said pensively that she did not know. So it was clear that a further need was:

• to understand what complications of diabetes may affect her, especially in relation to menstruation/ fertility/childbearing

Asked what she knew about possible ways of preventing the onset of any of the complications of diabetes, Kate displayed inadequate knowledge. She knew, in general, that it was important to avoid infection but was not knowledgeable about how to do so. This therefore could be considered another learning need:

• to gain knowledge of infection and its prevention

It became clear that since leaving school and starting work as a telephonist, Kate's way of life had altered considerably and some of the difficulties in controlling her diabetes seemed to arise directly from such changes.

While at school Kate's diet had been easy to regulate and her mother had supervised this closely. Now Kate ate in the canteen at work and found it less easy to control her food intake. In recent months she had put on a considerable amount of weight and had been unsuccessful in trying to reverse this situation. She was also going out a lot more and, as a result drank beer fairly regularly. Kate had not appreciated that beer had to be accounted for within her daily carbohydrate intake.

Three areas of teaching appeared to be required:
• review diet in the light of changed eating habits
• understand the significance of alcohol in the diet
• understand the importance of and how to achieve weight reduction

Mobilising was another AL which had altered since leaving school and starting work. Kate was now fairly inactive at work and had not continued any of the sports she pursued at school. She agreed there was a need:

• to review exercise habits/requirements

All the learning needs identified are listed together below. It is unlikely that the amount of re-education needed for this girl, who has been diabetic since a young age, would have been appreciated had there not been a thorough nursing assessment of this patient.

ALs	Learning needs identified
Maintaining a safe environment	Gain knowledge of infection and its prevention
Communicating	Reconsider, in the light of growing up, what being diabetic means
Eating and drinking	Review diet in the light of changed eating habits
	Understand the significance of alcohol in the diet
	Understand the importance of and how to achieve weight reduction
Mobilising	Review exercise habits/requirements
Expressing sexuality	Understand what complications of diabetes may affect her, especially in relation to menstruation/fertility/childbearing

Patient Assessment Form

Date of admission *10 April*   Date of assessment *10 April*

Surname   *WARRENDER*   Forenames *Kate*

Male   [ ]   Age [*17 6/12*]   Single/~~Married~~/~~Widowed~~ ✓   Prefers to be addressed as
Female [✓]   Other

Date of birth   *Kate*

Address of usual residence   *18 Kirkwood Crescent,*
Ballgreen Estate,
Newtown

Type of accommodation   *Semidetached house; 3 bedrooms and bathroom; garden.*

Family/Others at this residence   *Parents, brothers (20 and 16), sister (12)*

Next of kin   Name *Mr Keith Warrender*   Address *as above*

Relationship *Father*   Tel. no.   *063-8468*

Significant others   Relatives/~~Dependents~~ *family, as above*

Helpers

Visitors

Occupation   *Telephonist (since leaving school 18 months ago).*

Religious beliefs and relevant practices   *None*

Patient's perception of current health status   *Thinks that current imbalance of her diabetes was caused by infected toe.*

Reason for admission/~~referral~~   *Diabetic ketoacidosis*

Medical diagnosis

Past medical history   *Diagnosed as having diabetes when aged 8.*
Four admissions to hospital in ketoacidosis in past 18 months.

Allergies   *None*   Significant life crises

Fig. 5.1 Kate Warrender: assessment of ALs

Assessment of Activities of Living

Date *11 April*

Patient's problems
(actual/potential)
(p) = potential

AL	Usual routines: what he/she can and cannot do independently
● Maintaining a safe environment	Knows how to inject insulin safely. Knows she has to guard against infection but lacks knowledge of why and how.
● Communicating	Pleasant manner; enjoys talking about self and family; good vocabulary. No sensory impairment. Conveys anxiety about current problems.
● Breathing	Respiration, pulse, BP all within range of normal.
● Eating and drinking	Adheres to dietary modification because of diabetes- uses an 'exchange' system for diet. Finds canteen lunches difficult to incorporate in diet (used to take packed lunch to school). Has gained weight in recent months. Recently has begun to drink alcohol in evenings.
● Eliminating	Passes urine × 8 daily. Is confident about urine testing. Bowels regular (every other day).
● Personal cleansing and dressing	Enjoys grooming and fashionable dressing. Showers most evenings. Cleans teeth morning and night. Washes hair × 3 weekly.
● Controlling body temperature	Slightly pyrexial on admission (37·8°c)
● Mobilising	Used to be active / play sport at school; now has little exercise. Goes to work by bus and gets a lift home by car.
● Working and playing	Telephonist since leaving school - enjoys the job. No active hobbies now. Spare time is devoted to going to pub or cinema with boyfriend and friends.
● Expressing sexuality	Last menstruated 3 months ago and is worried because has not done so since. Seems uncertain about heredity / fertility aspects of diabetes.
● Sleeping	Usually sleeps well, except when worried. Shares bedroom with young sister. Bedtime irregular, often late. Uses duvet, 1 pillow.
● Dying	

6

Setting goals for evaluation

Having identified the patient's problems, the next step in the 'planning' phase of the process of nursing is to set goals—to decide what is to be achieved in the course of attempting to alleviate, solve or prevent the stated problems, actual and potential.

Setting specific goals is one of the activities which individualises and personalises nursing. Two patients may have the same problem but the appropriate goal for each is likely to be different. For example a young man confined to bed because of an injury to his spine has the potential problem of developing pressure sores. So too, does a very old lady who is in the final stages of terminal illness. But, whereas the goal for the young man would be:
- prevention of pressure sores

a more appropriate goal for the old lady would be:
- minimal movement/maximum comfort

TABLE 6.1 GOALS FOR NURSING UNCONSCIOUS PATIENTS

AL	Assessment	Problems
Maintaining a safe environment	Inactive protective reflexes which permit safe interaction with environment	Cannot blink bacteriolytic tears over conjunctiva; may dry and become infected
	The means of processing sensory input and responding to them is inactive	Cannot move away from pressure, heat, cold or any skin irritant
	Is there uncooperativeness/aggression?	Cannot hear, see, smell or move away from danger potential: may injure self or others
Communicating	The means of communicating verbally and non-verbally is inactive	Cannot make needs known
		Cannot communicate any discomfort
		There is evidence that some unconscious patients can hear and are aware of what is going on in their vicinity but are unable to communicate that they have received the sensory input (but may recall subsequently)

Whatever the goal, it must be a realistic target, it must be unambiguously stated and the time by which it is expected to be achieved should be specified.

Setting goals is not only important as the basis for planning relevant intervention, it is necessary if the evaluation phase of the process of nursing is to be carried out. Evaluation is only possible if the criteria for evaluation are pre-determined. An example of setting goals for evaluation is shown in the following presentation of a nursing plan for an unconscious patient.

MS JENNY HALL   Age 22

Unconscious from head injury

Jenny Hall had been making the long journey from her home to that of her parents to begin a week's holiday with them. On a foggy stretch of motorway, her car was involved in a pile-up collision. Jenny was taken from her vehicle, virtually uninjured but unconscious, and transferred to a nearby hospital along with other victims of the crash.

Three weeks later Jenny is still unconscious, but she has not developed any of the possible complications which may arise from head injury. Patients may remain unconscious for as long as this and yet, in the end, make a good recovery.

SETTING GOALS FOR NURSING

The broad objectives when nursing patients who are unconscious are to sustain their vital functions until they are able to do so, ensure their safe return to consciousness, and restore their independence in the ALs. One of the important factors about using the process of nursing is that it helps nurses to break down broad objectives like these into specific ones—*goals*.

A nursing plan showing the range of goals involved when nursing an unconscious patient—this state rendering the person totally dependent on others for the maintenance of all activities of living—is shown in tabular form below. The sort of problems involved, both actual and potential, have been identified and they are listed. The goals that might be set in relation to each problem have been worked out and their relevance to evaluation is demonstrated.

It is suggested that readers study each AL separately, in turn, in particular looking at the relationship between *goals* and *evaluation*.

Goals	Evaluation
Conjunctiva to remain moist and uninfected	Conjunctiva is moist and uninfected
Unblemished skin/no pressure sores	Skin is unblemished/no pressure sores
The patient will be unharmed	The patient is unharmed
Patient and staff will be unharmed	Patient and staff are unharmed
The patient will be unharmed physically and emotionally	No apparent discomfort/unmet need
All his needs will have been met	Patient communicates verbally and non-verbally
The patient will communicate verbally and non-verbally	Meaningful memories, if recall

TABLE 6.1 Continued

AL	Assessment	Problems
Breathing	Absent cough reflex Evidence of blood and/or vomit Position of lower jaw Breathing rate, depth, rhythm, sound, difficulty Colour of skin, cyanosis Pulse BP	Potential: airway obstruction, respiratory infection, pulmonary embolism
Eating and drinking	Absent swallowing reflex Large/medium/small body frame Height: Weight:	Cannot swallow Unsafe to feed orally Potential: dehydration, malnutrition, loss of weight
Eliminating	Bladder: full/empty/incontinence Bowel: full/empty/impacted/incontinence	Loss of voluntary control of anal and urethral sphincters Potential: excoriated skin, loss of tone in bladder, urinary infection, retention of urine, bladder stones, constipation, impacted faeces
Personal cleansing and dressing	Clothes, skin, hands and nails, hair, mouth and teeth	Total dependence for all activities incorporated in personal cleansing and dressing Potential: pressure sores, matted hair, dirty mouth, dental caries
Controlling body temperature	Measure temperature rectally Skin: colour; hot or cold to touch; moist or dry	Potential: dehydration from excess fluid loss through skin Weight loss from increased metabolic rate Abnormally high/low body temperature
Mobilising	Body alignment Describe any movement which the patient makes	Total dependence for positioning and moving any part of body Potential: muscle wasting; joint adhesions; contracures; deformity

Working and playing	Usual working activities
	Usual playing activities
		Potential: long absence from work;
		     may not be able to resume previous occupation;
		     may not be able to carry out some of previous hobbies

Goals	*Evaluation*
Breathing ⎫ Pulse ⎬ maintained at previous status/ within range of normal BP ⎭	Breathing ⎫ Pulse ⎬ at previous status/ within range of normal BP ⎭
Average weight relevant to age, height and physique	Average weight relevant to age, height and physique
Non-excoriated skin Excreting urine as before unconscious Clear urine of characteristic odour Bladder not distended more than capacity to trigger micturition Deposit-free urine Defaecation at individual's habitual frequency Presence of only soft faeces in rectum	Non-excoriated skin Urine clear and of characteristic odour No palpable bladder distension No urinary discomfort/infection Defaecating according to previous satisfactory habit
Clean, odour-free unblemished skin; no pressure sores Clean unmatted hair Moist, clean, odour-free mouth Undeteriorated dental status Well-groomed appearance	Unblemished skin; no pressure sores Clean well-groomed hair Moist clean odour-free mouth Undeteriorated dental status Well-groomed appearance
Maintenance of hydration Average weight relevant to age, height and physique Return of body temperature to within patient's range of normal	No evidence of dehydration Previous satisfactory weight Body temperature within range of normal
Good body alignment Return of ability to move all parts of the body Absence of deformity	Good body alignment Can move all parts of the body No deformity
Rehabilitation to previous occupation and hobbies	Able to resume previous occupation and hobbies *or* changed employment, changed hobbies

TABLE 6.1 Continued

AL	Assessment	Problems
Expressing sexuality	Menstruation	Having intimate parts of the body touched by strangers without the patient being able to give permission Dependence
Sleeping	Differentiate sleeping/unconsciousness Level of consciousness assessed by using Glasgow coma scale	Potential: too frequent disturbance Coma
Dying	Vital signs/signs of approaching death	Potential: death

INDIVIDUALISING THE GENERAL NURSING PLAN

The general nursing plan shown above could be used as the basis of an individualised nursing plan, suitable for a particular patient. Among other details pertaining to the individual patient, specific dates by which the goals are to be achieved could be added to the plan.

As an example of how the general plan was individualised for Jenny, two ALs will be discussed: *maintaining a safe environment* and *eating and drinking*.

Information about Jenny's ALs was obtained from her parents. They had come to the hospital the morning after the accident, naturally shocked and anxious. They kept in close contact with the hospital throughout Jenny's time there. As their daughter lived in her own flat now, they were not aware of some details concerning some of her ALs. The information they provided is shown in Jenny's Patient Assessment Form (Fig. 6.1). Later, additional data were collected from friends who visited her.

AL of maintaining a safe environment. The first two items in the assessment column of the general plan applied to Jenny and there is always the possibility that patients returning to consciousness will be uncooperative and aggressive. The first three problems were identified from her nursing assessment data and the possibility of the fourth problem had to be borne in mind. Setting a goal for each of Jenny's identified problems permitted a weekly date to be added to the items in the column headed 'goals' in the table. Evaluation took place each week and so far the goals have been achieved.

AL of eating and drinking. Jenny's nursing assessment data revealed an absent swallowing reflex, that she was tall 1.8 m (5ft 10in), of medium body frame and well nourished 63.5 kg (weight 10 st.). Her parents supplied the information that she normally eats well, takes a varied diet and only drinks alcohol socially.

Jenny's identified eating and drinking problems were therefore as in the general plan. Because she could not swallow, it was unsafe to feed orally so that there were three potential problems: dehydration, malnutrition and loss of weight. Setting the goals for these problems was straightforward—to maintain her weight at 63.5 kg. and again a weekly date was attached to the goal and to the evaluation. However, subjective evidence that Jenny was not losing weight was accepted, as weighing was not considered desirable. So far the parenteral feeding regime is evaluated as achieving the set goal, for Jenny does not appear to have lost weight. Should this occur the nutritional content of her diet would be re-assessed.

AN ASSESSMENT/EVALUATION TOOL

It cannot be too strongly stressed that the same tool can be used for assessment and evaluation. Assessment is collecting data by measurement and/or observation and examination. The same activities are carried out in evaluation and the collected data are evaluated against the stated goals or patient outcomes to discover whether or not the goals have been achieved.

An assessment/evaluation tool referred to in the general nursing plan for unconscious patients is the Glasgow coma scale (see Table 6.2). Jenny's score was 6 so that she was correctly referred to as a 'comatose' patient. The scale has been tested for reliability and validity and is recommended as a reliable assessment/evaluation tool when nursing comatose patients.

Goals	Evaluation
Prevention of psychological upset on return to consciousness Clean odour-free perineum	No apparent psychological upset Clean odour-free perineum
Minimum disturbance to patient; return to consciousness	Patient disturbed only when necessary Response to the criteria in the Glasgow coma scale
Prevent unnecessary death; promote peaceful dying	Continues to live; dies peacefully

TABLE 6.2 GLASGOW COMA SCALE

	Eye opening *Score*	Motor response *Score*	Verbal response *Score*
high score		6 If command such as 'lift up your hands' is obeyed	
		5 If purposeful movement to remove painful stimulus such as pressure over eyebrow	5 If oriented to person, place and time
	4 If eyes open spontaneously to approach of nurse to bedside	4 If finger withdrawn after application of painful stimulus to it	4 If conversation confused
	3 If eyes open in response to speech	3 If painful stimulation at finger tip flexes the elbow	3 If inappropriate words are used
	2 If eyes open in response to pain at finger tip	2 If the patient's arms are flexed and finger tip stimulation results in extension of elbow	2 If only incomprehensible sounds are uttered
low score	1 If eyes do not open in response to pain at finger tip	1 If there is no detectable response to repeated and various stimuli	1 If no verbal response

A normal person would score 15 on the scale; the lowest possible score is 3 which is compatible with, but does not necessarily indicate, brain death. A score of 7 is used as a definition of coma.

REFERENCE

Teasdale G 1975 Assessing 'conscious level'. Nursing Times 71 (24) June 12: 914–917

Patient Assessment Form

Date of admission *18 February*

Date of assessment *18 February*

Surname **HALL**

Forenames *Jennifer*

Male ☐
Female ☑

Age **22**

Date of birth

Single ✓ /Married/Widowed
Other

Prefers to be addressed as

Jenny

Address of usual residence *2 St Andrew's Square, Scotstown*

Type of accommodation *2-apartment flat*

Family/Others at this residence *None. Lives alone.*

Next of kin
Name *Mr Clive Hall*
Relationship *Father*

Address *The Courts Manfield Meadows Berwick-upon-sea*
Tel. no. *737-0693*

Significant others

Relatives/Dependents *Mother and father (no siblings)*

Helpers

Visitors *Occasional visits from parents; friend (Ann Black) and boyfriend (Neil Bayley) from Scotstown*

Occupation *Bank Clerk*

Religious beliefs and relevant practices *Church of England*

Patient's perception of current health status *Patient unconscious*

Reason for admission/referral *Road traffic accident - unconscious*

Medical diagnosis *Head injury: unconscious*

Past medical history *Nil of note*

Allergies *None*

Significant life crises *None*

Fig. 6.1 Jennifer Hall: assessment of ALs

Assessment of Activities of Living

AL | Usual routines:
what he/she can and cannot do independently

● Maintaining
a safe
environment

Usually a careful driver ; no previous accidents.

● Communicating

Has good sight and hearing. Is well educated and articulate; good vocabulary; is not shy.

● Breathing

Does not smoke. Has not had recent cold or cough. On admission, breathing deep and 18 per minute; pulse 70.

● Eating and
drinking

Normally eats well; varied diet, no particular likes/dislikes. Tall (height 5'10"); medium body frame; weight 10 stone.

● Eliminating

*No problems known to parents, friends.
Was incontinent of urine at site of accident.*

● Personal
cleansing and
dressing

Usually very well groomed and dressed. Clean and hair clean on admission.

● Controlling
body
temperature

On admission, temperature 37.2°C. Skin warm to the touch, normal colour; no excessive perspiration.

● Mobilising

No problems. Usually active and fit.

● Working
and playing

Apparently enjoys her job and is ambitious to progress. Hobbies include skiing and sailing.

● Expressing
sexuality

Was menstruating at time of admission.

● Sleeping

No difficulties known.

● Dying

7

Selecting appropriate nursing intervention

In the planning phase of the process of nursing, once goals are set, the appropriate nursing intervention to achieve these goals must be decided and written in unambiguous terms on the nursing plan.

In a study of communication among nurses, Lelean (1973) found that many traditionally much-used statements of nursing action were ambiguous. For example she describes one ward where the terms 'up for short periods' and 'up for long periods' were used. The first term meant between one and three hours for 43 per cent of the patients while for 57 per cent it meant up for longer than three hours. 'Up for long periods' also meant up for longer than three hours, although for 68 per cent of the patients it meant up for six hours or more. This shows clearly the need to describe nursing activities unambiguously (for example in the above instructions, to specify the time) when using nursing plans.

Another required skill is the ability to select from the range of nursing activities relevant to a particular patient's problem, the appropriate nursing intervention. Some problems may not be amenable to nursing help and, in such cases, the nursing activity selected will be referral to the appropriate agency or professional group.

To illustrate the activity of selecting appropriate nursing intervention and demonstrate how selected activities are stated on the nursing plan, Mr Hamilton, a patient with a variety of problems related to one AL—mobilising—has been chosen.

MR JOHN F. HAMILTON   Age 60
Problems with the
AL of mobilising

Mr Hamilton had a long history of a 'valvular heart condition' which probably accounted for his statement on admission that he had never been an active man. But twelve years ago he experienced, temporarily, total dependence for the AL of mobilising when he suffered a myocardial infarction. Since then his status on the dependence/independence continuum for mobilising has ranged from shorter periods of total dependence in hospital for major surgery, to longer periods at home and work at his optimal level, which over time became increasingly limited. Mr Hamilton's changing status on the dependence/independence continuum is illustrated in Figure 7.1 which shows that for two months before the current admission for a left below knee amputation he had been almost totally dependent for mobilising. He was housebound and could only shuffle about hanging on to furniture; he had been suffering excruciating pain in the left foot, sometimes even at rest; the left big toe and the adjacent one were gangrenous, so Mr Hamilton was admitted to hospital.

ASSESSMENT ON ADMISSION

Mr Hamilton looked ill, in pain, and older than his sixty years. After he had had time to recover from the journey the admission nursing assessment was carried out. Most of the biographical and health data on the left-hand side of the Patient Assessment Form (Fig. 7.2) were collected from Mr Hamilton's case notes. The data about activities of living on the right-hand side show clearly what a widespread effect the dependence for mobilising had on Mr Hamilton's other ALs. He was afraid of falling because he could not put his full weight on his painful left foot; he communicated his worry about his ill health, particularly about the immediate problem of his left foot. He attributed his loss of weight and poor appetite to lack of exercise, and due to limitation on mobilising he had had to retire prematurely at 59. Without doubt he needed nursing help in relation to his current limited mobilising resulting from his painful left foot.

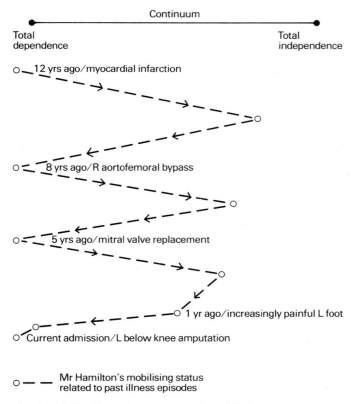

Continuum

Total dependence   Total independence

○—12 yrs ago/myocardial infarction

○—8 yrs ago/R aortofemoral bypass

○—5 yrs ago/mitral valve replacement

○—1 yr ago/increasingly painful L foot

○—Current admission/L below knee amputation

○ — — Mr Hamilton's mobilising status related to past illness episodes

Fig. 7.1 Mr Hamilton: changing status for mobilising

DEPENDENCE FOR MOBILISING: PAINFUL FOOT

Examination of Mr Hamilton's left foot revealed that the skin over the whole foot was a blotchy purple colour and almost all of the big toe and a third of the adjacent toe were black. Atherosclerosis (hardening and narrowing of the arteries) resulted in the deficient blood supply causing the appearance of Mr Hamilton's left foot. Raising the head of the bed is likely to assist blood supply to the feet. Deficiency of blood renders tissue vulnerable to infection and so foot hygiene is a preventive nursing activity. Placing a bedcradle over the feet falls into this preventive category because it relieves pressure from bedclothes on already damaged tissue. Turning the bedclothes over the cradle to leave the foot exposed permits frequent observation without disturbing an ill patient; it also helps to keep the foot cool, and cool tissue needs less oxygen; lastly it permits evaporation of perspiration which not only assists in cooling, but in Mr Hamilton's case prevents the damaged tissue becoming 'soggy'. These appropriate nursing interventions can be written on the plan as follows:

- raise head of bed
- foot hygiene
- bedcradle over feet
- turn bedclothes back to expose left foot
- observe left foot hourly

As a result of the excruciating pain in Mr Hamilton's left foot the doctor had prescribed an analgesic drug to be given 4 hourly when necessary. After discussion with Mr Hamilton the first dose was given immediately and thereafter regularly four hourly in anticipation of the fact that the pain was unlikely to abate in such badly damaged tissue. An additional appropriate nursing intervention on the plan was:

- pain control by 4 hourly administration of prescribed analgesic

By early evening Mr Hamilton had consented to have a below knee amputation the next day, but it was obvious he still had many reservations. However, the appropriate nursing intervention at this point was to revise the general pre- and postoperative regime and its rationale with him before talking specifically about amputation (he had had major surgery on two previous occasions).

The ward policy was to talk to patients before amputation explaining how in early life the brain receives sensory information from the rest of the body from which it constructs a 'map', often called the 'body image'. As this image is an important part of dignity and self-esteem, it is perfectly natural for a person to react emotionally to amputation because it is a direct assault on personal identity and integrity. Many emotions may be experienced: anger, aggression, denial, frustration, regression; emotions, as Murray Parkes (1975) points out, that are similar to those common in bereavement. The appropriate nursing intervention is to help patients to work through these feelings and use them constructively in the rehabilitation programme to help them achieve optimal mobilising.

Removal of the left foreleg would not produce immediate change in the brain's sensory map, so Mr Hamilton was made aware that after the operation he might feel that the leg was still intact; indeed he might experience pain in it—phantom pain.

The rehabilitative programme for a person who has had a lower amputation was also outlined for him. By being familiar with the postoperative nursing plan, and aware of his necessary involvement in it, he could begin to rebuild his confidence. These appropriate nursing interventions were summarised on the nursing plan:

- psychological preparation for amputation
- preparation for rehabilitation

DEPENDENCE FOR MOBILISING: BELOW KNEE STUMP

Mr Hamilton's chronic chest infection (see Fig. 7.2—AL of breathing) played a part in the selection of appropriate nursing interventions related to mobilising in the first four postoperative days. He was nursed in the sitting position for more effective coughing, so measures had to be taken to prevent flexion deformity of the left knee and to maintain

Patient Assessment Form

Date of admission *20 November*   Date of assessment *20 November*

Surname *HAMILTON*   Forenames *John Ferguson*

Male [✓]   Age [*60*]   ~~Single~~/Married[✓]/~~Widowed~~   Prefers to be addressed as
Female [ ]   Other   *Mr Hamilton*

Date of birth

Address of usual residence *3 Waterford Court*
Newtown

Type of accommodation *Two-storey terraced house. Bathroom. Additional W.C. downstairs.*

Family/Others at this residence *Wife*

Next of kin   Name *Mrs Jane Hamilton*   Address *as above*
     Relationship *Wife*   Tel. no. *063 2828*

Significant others   Relatives/~~Dependents~~ *2 sons (both married with young children)*

     Helpers

     Visitors

Occupation *Retired book binder (retired 1 yr ago on health grounds)*

Religious beliefs and relevant practices *Church of Scotland: wishes visit from hospital chaplain.*

Patient's perception of current health status *Understands amputation is likely to be necessary.*

Reason for admission/~~referral~~ *Severe pain/gangrene in L foot.*

Medical diagnosis *P.V.D. Gangrene in big and adjacent toe of L foot.*

Past medical history *Myocardial infarction 12 yrs ago; R aortofemoral bypass 8 yrs ago; mitral valve replacement 5 yrs ago; acute bronchitis 3 yrs ago.*

Allergies *Aspirin*   Significant life crises *Retired a year ago.*

Fig. 7.2 Mr Hamilton: assessment with problems stated

Assessment of Activities of Living

Date 20/21 Nov

AL	Usual routines: what he/she can and cannot do independently	Patient's problems (actual/potential) (p) = potential
● Maintaining a safe environment	Has been feeling more at risk of falling as pain in L foot has increased, causing limited mobility.	● Feels at risk of falling
● Communicating	Does not hear well; more deaf in L ear than R ear. Sight good. Says he is a quiet person. Conveys anxiety about current admission and says he is weary with his prolonged ill health.	● Poor hearing (L ear) ● Worried about admission/ill health
● Breathing	Has a cough; expectorates green sputum. Often feels breathless. On admission, respirations 22/min; pulse 108; BP 110/98	● Cough ● Infected sputum
● Eating and drinking	Poor appetite because of prolonged illness, pain and lack of exercise/fresh air. Has lost weight over recent years; is very thin.	● Poor appetite ● Loss of weight
● Eliminating	Passes urine x 4-6 daily. Bowels regular (every day or two). Uses a stick to help himself rise from WC.	
● Personal cleansing and dressing	Washes a.m. and p.m.; shaves a.m.; baths once every fortnight or so, with assistance from wife. Has dentures. No evidence of pressure sores. Gangrenous L foot.	● Gangrenous L foot ● (p) Pressure sores
● Controlling body temperature	Temperature on admission 38.2°C. Feels warm, perspiring.	● Discomfort from raised body temperature
● Mobilising	Difficulty with mobilising due to pain in L foot. Increasingly housebound over last year.	● Difficulty with walking ● Pain in L foot
● Working and playing	Retired prematurely due to ill-health. Now unable to pursue active hobbies. Watches TV; reads newspapers, thrillers. Misses work.	● Anxiety about premature retirement
● Expressing sexuality	Has expressed anxiety about his enforced dependence on his wife and says this and his retirement has made him feel he has lost his masculinity.	● Feeling of loss of masculinity due to dependence.
● Sleeping	Sleeps very poorly, disturbed by pain and worry.	● Poor sleeper
● Dying		

ability to move his left hip. Deep breathing and right foot exercises were encouraged hourly to prevent pulmonary embolism. For the first few days, Mr Hamilton needed help with the mobilising aspects of the AL of personal cleansing and dressing (including a bed bath and measures to prevent pressure sores) and also with the AL of eliminating (using a urinal/bedpan). All of these nursing interventions were summarised thus on his nursing plan:

- maintain sitting position; encourage coughing, expectoration
- prevent flexion deformity of left knee
- maintain ability to move left hip
- deep breathing and right foot exercises hourly
- help with mobilising aspects of personal cleansing and dressing (bed bath; prevention of pressure sores);
- help with eliminating (urinal/bedpan)

With the help of the physiotherapist and a nurse, Mr Hamilton was transferred from bed to chair for bedmaking on the first two postoperative days. As it is important to re-establish the sense of balance in preparation for mobilising, Mr Hamilton was encouraged to stand for one minute with arms supported on his helpers' shoulders each time he got out of and back into bed. By the third day, he felt well enough to attempt early standing by having a metal pylon with a foot attachment fixed to the metal socket which had been embedded in the plaster cast surrounding the stump. Another nursing intervention was therefore to observe the stump frequently for any sign of pressure or friction sore and to be on the alert for pain under the mould, elevated temperature and foul smell—all possible manifestations of a stump sore.

On the fourth postoperative day and thereafter, Mr Hamilton was taught press-ups and weight-bearing on hands, while sitting, with the objective of strengthening the shoulder girdle muscles in preparation for crutch walking. He was also taught thigh-lifting from the bed, and flexion/extension of both knees to strengthen the muscles required for eventually walking with a prosthesis. The nursing intervention, therefore, was supervising these exercises.

The stump mould was removed on the seventh day so the pylon weight-bearing was changed to crutch weight-bearing taught by the physiotherapist. She instructed that Mr Hamilton's energy level would be the guide as to the distance walked. Because of Mr Hamilton's poor circulation and chest and heart condition, it was important to prevent undue exhaustion now that he was feeling better than he had done for some months.

Another nursing intervention during the second week was to teach stump care: removal and re-application of a firm bandage twice daily to ensure a cone-shaped stump ready for the prosthesis. Toughening of the stump was achieved by laying a pillow on a stool on to which the stump was placed with increasing pressure.

By the third week, the main nursing intervention was

helping Mr Hamilton to adjust to the idea that now his 'work' was looking after himself even if it took most of the day. Although his mobilising ability increased with his improving general condition, his poor circulation only permitted him to carry out everyday living activities if he took his time.

The many appropriate nursing interventions directly related to the walking aspects of the AL of mobilising during Mr Hamilton's stay in hospital are summarised below:

Postoperative Day	Nursing intervention
1	transfer to chair for bedmaking; standing; observe stump
2	transfer to chair for one hour; standing; observe stump
3	early standing with pylon; observe stump
4 5 6	encourage/supervise: press-ups, weight-bearing on hands while sitting, thigh-lifting, flexion/extension both knees — observe stump ×6 daily
7	as 4, 5, 6 + remove stump mould; no pylon; observe stump ×6 daily
8 ... 14	as 4, 5, 6 + start crutch walking with physiotherapist; energy level to guide distance walked, avoid exhaustion; teach stump care; remove, re-apply firm bandage ×2 daily; pillow on stool for weight-bearing ×2 daily
15 21	continue + adjust to idea that looking after self is now 'work' (discharge to care of GP and District Nurse. Outpatient appointment in 6 weeks)

All of the nursing interventions mentioned in this section were selected to help Mr Hamilton to overcome mobilising problems. As the nature of the problem with the AL of mobilising altered, so too did the type of nursing intervention selected.

This section also demonstrates the usefulness of looking at one AL in relation to the concept of a dependence/independence continuum. In the introduction it was shown how the patient's status on the continuum had changed over the years prior to this admission to hospital. The remainder of the section shows the changes during the pre- and post-operative phases of his stay.

Although the rationale for each intervention mentioned in the above list has to be looked for in the text, this section does demonstrate that whatever nursing interventions are selected, they can be written succinctly on the nursing plan—even when the patient has several complications.

REFERENCES

Lelean S 1973 Ready for report nurse? Royal College of Nursing, London, p 69
Murray Parkes C 1975 Reaction to the loss of a limb. Nursing Mirror 140 1 January 2: 36–40

8

Recording nursing intervention

In Chapter 7, the activity of selecting appropriate nursing interventions was discussed, and the conclusion reached that it is possible to include detail of all appropriate activities in a written nursing plan. However, in addition, there must be some record of the activities actually implemented for that patient. In other words, in addition to preselection and statement of a plan, *recording nursing interventions* is necessary.

There are a number of reasons why this recording is important, in addition to the most obvious one of confirming that the planned intervention was indeed carried out. *When* it was carried out and *by which nurse* may be important factors to record. And, if the plan was *not* implemented, the reason why may be crucial information for subsequent planning. It is also essential, if evaluation is to be undertaken properly, to be sure what intervention was carried out. In the long-term, written nursing plans and records of the interventions could provide nursing's data base; the accumulated data from many patients could be analysed to show the effectiveness (or ineffectiveness) of specific nursing activities, and to improve understanding of the complexities of nursing.

So, plans alone are not enough: records of the implementation of the plan must be maintained alongside. To illustrate how this may be done, this section shows how nursing activities, implemented to help a patient admitted for a gastroscopy, were recorded.

MR BOB JONES   Age 43

Admitted for gastroscopy

For 20 years Mr Jones had endured attacks of indigestion which gradually became worse. He was aware that he had 'ulcer trouble'. He worried in case the ulcer would burst when he was driving his lorry on the motorway resulting in him lying bleeding at the roadside before help came. His doctor continued to advise him that he should have hospital treatment for this condition but his anxiety about the prospect of going into hospital—perhaps for an operation—was so intense that he pleaded to continue his 'medical' treatment under the family doctor. His anxiety was part of a vicious circle that prevented the ulcer healing: to overcome his 'nerves', he generally smoked cigarettes and drank alcohol in excess but when the pain was so bad that it terrified him, he smoked and drank even more; a stressful job, irregular meals and a poor diet completed the vicious circle.

However, recently, he had been off sick for five months and missed the extra money he earned in full employment, particularly as his three children were at an age when they needed more money. He himself was bored, and the pain was not improving with the additional rest. So he agreed at last to a hospital investigation (gastroscopy), possibly to be followed by surgery.

ASSESSMENT

Mr Jones had a pleasant manner and an uninhibited way of talking to the nurse while she collected the biographical and health data (Fig. 8.1). He was very frank while giving information about his ALs, from which he agreed that he had several health problems. These are written on the right-hand side of the form.

PLANNING

Mr Jones showed considerable interest in his health problems and was determined as he said 'to mend his ways'. So it was considered worth writing in the plan (Table 8.1) some long-term goals for his problems of obesity, excessive

Patient Assessment Form

Date of admission *23 October*   Date of assessment *23 October*

Surname *JONES*   Forenames *Robert (Bob)*

Male ✓   Age *43*   Single̶/Married/̶W̶i̶d̶o̶w̶e̶d̶   Prefers to be addressed as
Female ☐   Other   *Mr Jones*
                      Date of birth

Address of usual residence *6 Challerton Road,*
                            Longhill

Type of accommodation *Small terraced house, with bathroom*

Family/Others at this residence *Wife and 3 children (aged 16, 12, 8)*

Next of kin   Name *Mrs Mary Jones*   Address *as above*

               Relationship *Wife*   Tel. no. *028 91069*

Significant others   Relatives/Dependents ⎫ *wife, 3 children*

                      Helpers   ⎬

                      Visitors   ⎭

Occupation *Heavy goods vehicle driver*

Religious beliefs and relevant practices *Church of England*

Patient's perception of current health status *Knows he may need surgery to treat ulcer.*

Reason for admission/r̶e̶f̶e̶r̶r̶a̶l̶ *Gastroscopy.*

Medical diagnosis *? Duodenal ulcer*

Past medical history *Indigestion and stomach pains for 20 years. Has been off work for past fu*
                      mon

Allergies *None*   Significant life crises

Fig. 8.1 Mr Jones: assessment with problems stated

Assessment of Activities of Living

Date *23 Oct*

AL	Usual routines: what he/she can and cannot do independently	Patient's problems (actual/potential) (p) = potential
● Maintaining a safe environment	Became concerned that ulcer might burst while driving his lorry.	● Anxiety when driving
● Communicating	Conveyed his intense anxiety about proposed investigation and probable operation on admission. Pleasant manner; uninhibited in talking to nurses.	● Excessive anxiety about investigation/ surgery
● Breathing	Smokes 40 cigarettes per day, more when anxious. Cough; dark sputum; occasional wheeze.	● Cough with sputum ● Smokes
● Eating and drinking	Overweight (83 kg; height 150 cm). Poor diet — irregular, frequent fried dishes. Eating relieves pain; milk also. Drinks excessively, especially weekends.	● Obesity ● Pain/water-brash ● Excessive alcohol consumption
● Eliminating	Passes urine x 3–5 daily, more at week-ends. Bowels regular (daily); occasional melaena.	
● Personal cleansing and dressing	Baths and shaves most days. Well groomed and dressed. Missing teeth and others rotten.	● Dental caries
● Controlling body temperature	Temperature 37°C on admission.	
● Mobilising	Full range of movement. Normally not very active.	
● Working and playing	Has lost a great deal of working time due to ulcer trouble. Off work for past 5 months due to pain and 'nerves'. Main leisure activity is drinking.	● Absence from work due to ill-health
● Expressing sexuality	Conveys desire to appear masculine; dislikes being helped to carry out ALS.	
● Sleeping	Goes to bed at midnight; gets up at variable time (0600–0930 hrs). When disturbed by waterbrash, sleeps sitting up. Does not take sleeping pills.	● Sleep disturbed by pain/ waterbrash
● Dying		

TABLE 8.1 MR JONES: NURSING PLAN

AL	Problem	Goal	Nursing intervention	Evaluation
Maintaining a safe environment	Excessive health anxiety when driving lorry	Drive without health anxiety	Use his expressed anxiety to motivate cooperation	
Communicating	Excessive anxiety about gastroscopy and possible surgery	Decreased anxiety	Check, wear identiband; discover what he knows about investigation and operation; correct erroneous information; give needed information	

Breathing	Cough with sputum	Decreased coughing
		Lessened sputum
			No smoking
			  stay away from smoking areas
			  chat with non-smoking patients
			  use motivators frequently
			  praise abstinence
			
			Deep breathing and coughing × 8 daily
			
			Observing, measuring sputum daily	

	Smokes at least 40 high tar cigs daily	Smoking no more than 20 medium tar cigs daily (Mr Jones does not want to give up smoking completely)	Help identify when he experiences stress → smoking Help plan when he will smoke the 20 cigs; praise for keeping to plan; help him develop other ways of coping with stress	
Eating and drinking	Modification of diet	Clear visualisation of gastric lining; prevention of malnourishment	Low residue lunch, supper Milky drink 22.00 Nil by mouth/swallow reflex +	
	Obesity/ Excessive alcohol consumption	Taking 4500 kJ diet Improved eating habits Drinking no more than 2 whiskies daily	Teach dangers of obesity Discuss acceptable low kilojoule diet Weight/alcohol chart Praise weight loss Use safe driving as motivator	
	Pain Water-brash	Relief from surgery	Pre- and postoperative nursing	
Personal cleansing and dressing	Dental caries	Improved dental hygiene Dental appointment	Teach dangers of dental caries; mouth cleaning after meals; necessity for dental appointment	
	(p) pressure sore	No pressure sore	Norton scoring scale	

TABLE 8.1 Continued

AL	Problem	Goal	Nursing intervention	Evaluation
Mobilising	p = DVT	No DVT	Remain ambulant today Lower limb exercises to prevent DVT	
Working and playing	Absence from work due to ill-health	Return to work minus health anxiety (less alcohol)	Use driving without health anxiety as motivator	
Sleeping	Sleep disturbed by pain, water-brash, enforced sitting up	Sleep lying down without pain	One sleeping pill 22.00	

smoking and alcohol consumption. His graphic description of feeling terrified that the ulcer would burst while he was driving was to be used as a motivator to help him cooperate in carrying out the plan.

RECORDING NURSING INTERVENTION

The nursing plan to help Mr Jones cope with his health problems related to the *AL of communicating*—excessive anxiety about gastroscopy and possible surgery—required to be implemented on the first day. The nurse responsible for Mr Jones filled in the record sheet as follows:

Date	AL	Record of nursing intervention	Initials	Time
23/10	Communicating	Checked identiband, worn; seems reassured that he knows what to expect at gastroscopy	AH	16.00

Close scrutiny of this reveals that there is now a written record of the date and time of the nursing intervention, by whom it was carried out, and Mr Jones's reaction to it.

The nursing plan to help Mr Jones cope with his health problems related to the *AL of breathing* involved the setting of priorities. The problem to be tackled immediately was how to get his lungs into the best possible condition should a general anaesthetic be necessary in a few days' time. He agreed not to smoke before the anaesthetic, so the planned nursing intervention was to advise and reinforce:

- staying away from the dayroom in which smoking was permitted
- chatting with other non-smoking patients
- using motivators frequently
    prevention of chest infection
    driving without health anxiety
- praising abstinence

It was imperative to clear Mr Jones's respiratory tract of at least some of the sputum causing wheeziness, so the appropriate planned interventions to be implemented immediately are:

- deep breathing and coughing × 8 daily
- observing, measuring sputum daily

The remainder of the nursing plan related to the AL of breathing was longer term policy as Mr Jones had enough to cope with, carrying out the selected planned activities, so below is a record of the implemented nursing interventions on the first day:

Date	AL	Record of nursing intervention	Initials	Time
23/10	Breathing	Not seen smoking	AH	14.15
		Deep breathing and coughing	AH	15.05
			AH	15.55
			AH	16.30
			AH	17.30
			AH	18.35
			AH	19.55
		30 ml greenish sputum	BA	22.00

A glance at Mr Jones's nursing plan related to the *AL of eating and drinking* reveals a problem of modification of diet, to low residue, in order to improve visibility of the gastric lining during investigation; the relevant nursing intervention is observation and recording of intake. To further improve gastric visibility Mr Jones will have nil by mouth after 22.00 hours; the fasting will be continued until the re-establishment of a safe swallowing reflex which will be disrupted by application of local anaesthetic to the pharyngeal wall immediately prior to gastroscopy. But to avoid even temporary malnourishment during the investigation, the nursing plan states that he will have a milky drink at 22.00 hours. But how will the staff know whether or not the plan has been carried out? Only if a record is kept of the nursing intervention as below:

Date	AL	Record of nursing intervention	Initials	Time
23/10	Eating and drinking	Ate low residue lunch	AB	12.30
		supper	AK	18.30
		Drank milky drink	BA	22.00
24/10		Nil by mouth/to endoscopy room	AB	10.00
		Swallowing reflex +	AK	14.00
		Cup of tea	AK	14.15
		Tea and ham sandwich	AK	14.30
		Low residue supper	AK	18.00
		Milky drink	BA	20.00

Again it was not appropriate to implement the remainder of the planned nursing interventions, as the decision was made to operate as soon as possible. So after surgery the intervention will be implemented and recorded.

Only if there is a problem with the *AL of eliminating* is bowel preparation necessary prior to gastroscopy. In spite of Mr Jones's poor diet and irregular hours of eating, at the assessment interview he said his bowels 'were regular as clockwork—every morning'. However, now that surgery is imminent the nursing plan will be updated to include pre-operative bowel preparation and related nursing interventions, and they will be recorded as they are implemented.

Sufficient has been said to demonstrate to the reader the rationale of recording nursing interventions and to illustrate the relevance of the nursing plan to the 'record of nursing intervention'. It is essential for nurses to realise the importance of these documents in providing a permanent record of nursing.

9

Using the process when nursing acutely ill patients

A common criticism of the process of nursing is that it is too complex and too time-consuming to be used when nursing acutely ill patients. Naturally, in an emergency, no-one expects the nurse to spend time drawing up a detailed nursing plan. However, that does not mean to say that the *process* cannot be employed.

In fact, in an emergency situation, it is crucial for the patient's problems to be correctly identified so that the most effective intervention is decided upon without wasting time. Frequent evaluation is essential to monitor the patient's response to the activities implemented and guide subsequent intervention. So, the process is used. The main difference in an emergency context is that progress through its phases is more rapid, the result being that the process is repeated again and again. Only absolutely crucial data, such as recordings of vital signs and drugs administered, are documented until time permits. Most important of all is that priorities must be determined: of the problems identified, only those which are considered to be life-threatening are dealt with initially.

Any severe difficulty with breathing is an obvious example of a life-threatening problem. The patient in this case, Mr Morton, was admitted as an emergency, with severe difficulty in breathing arising from an asthma attack.

MR WILLIAM MORTON   Age 40
Severe difficulty
in breathing

Mr Morton is a forty-year-old, self-employed greengrocer. He has suffered from chronic bronchitis since he was twenty-five and, until six years ago, smoked 40 cigarettes a day. Since then he has not smoked. However, he still has a morning cough which produces sputum; he is aware of wheeziness as he breathes and, over the last 15 years, has had a number of severe chest infections. Increasingly, he has become breathless on exertion. He is obese.

For three weeks he has been suffering from an acute respiratory infection and this has resulted in two very severe attacks of asthma. These were treated at home by the family doctor. However, a third attack did not respond to treatment, the bronchospasm remained and so severe was Mr Morton's breathing difficulty he was immediately admitted to hospital.

ASSESSMENT ON ADMISSION

Mr Morton was unable to breathe in the lying down position and so was brought to the ward from the casualty department in a wheelchair, supported in the upright sitting position. His difficulty in breathing was both visible and audible, the main observations from immediate assessment being:
- breathing wheezy and gasping
- lips blue, cheeks purple
- difficulty in talking
- looked exhausted and distressed

Two nurses lifted Mr Morton into bed, maintaining his sitting position. While the ward doctor examined the patient, one nurse attended to Mrs Morton who had accompanied her husband to hospital. She was able to provide most of the information which appears on the left-hand side of this patient's Assessment Form (Fig. 9.1).

THE PRIORITY PROBLEM: SEVERE BREATHLESSNESS

A number of nursing activities were implemented immediately in order to alleviate Mr Morton's breathing difficulty. These included:
- maintaining patient in upright sitting position
- administration of prescribed drugs

Patient Assessment Form

Date of admission *8 October*   Date of assessment *8 October*

Surname **MORTON**   Forenames *William*

Male [✓]   Age [40]   ~~Single~~/Married ✓/~~Widowed~~   Prefers to be addressed as
Female [ ]   Other :   *Mr Morton*
                  Date of birth

Address of usual residence   *17a Park Avenue*
                                  Broadmeadow.

Type of accommodation   *Small terraced cottage with W.C. and shower.*

Family/~~Others~~ at this residence   *Wife and 2 young children*

Next of kin   Name *Mrs Betty Morton*   Address *.as above*
                                                             No telephone. (Tel. no. of
                   Relationship *Wife*   Tel. no. *Broadmeadow police station is*
                                                                      890 3321)

Significant others   Relatives/Dependents *Wife and 2 children*

                          Helpers *If needed, mother-in-law*

                          Visitors *Above family members*

Occupation   *Self-employed greengrocer*

Religious beliefs and relevant practices   *Roman Catholic*

Patient's perception of current health status *Knows he has severe asthma attack due to infection*

Reason for admission/~~referral~~ *Emergency admission - severe breathlessness*

Medical diagnosis   *Status asthmaticus*

Past medical history   *Pneumonia in infancy.* *Chronic bronchitis since age 25.*
                                                      Has had acute respiratory infection past 3/52.

Allergies   *None known.*   Significant life crises

Fig. 9.1 Mr Morton: assessment with problems stated

Assessment of Activities of Living

Date *8 Oct*

AL	Usual routines: what he/she can and cannot do independently	Patient's problems (actual/potential) (p) = potential
● Maintaining a safe environment	Independent usually.	● Dependent
● Communicating	Usually communicative. No sensory impairment. On admission unable to talk due to breathlessness.	● Difficulty in talking. Distressed.
● Breathing	Usually has morning cough with sputum and breathlessness on exertion. Severe dyspnoea on admission; breathing wheezy and gasping.	● Severe difficulty in breathing.
● Eating and drinking	Overweight: according to wife, has high carbohydrate intake (including a lot of beer).	● Obesity. ● Dependent due to bedrest.
● Eliminating	No problems.	● Dependent due to bedrest.
● Personal cleansing and dressing	Showers, shaves, washes hair daily. Apparent dental caries.	● Dependent due to bedrest ● Dental caries
● Controlling body temperature	Always has higher than normal temperature when suffering from chest infection. Temperature 38·4°C on admission.	● Pyrexia
● Mobilising	Full range of movement. Tends to limit activity to avoid breathlessness. On admission, unable to breathe lying down.	● Dependent due to bedrest ● Unable to lie down.
● Working and playing	Self-employed greengrocer. Job takes up most of the time. Watching TV is major relaxation.	● Anxiety because absent from work.
● Expressing sexuality	Nil of relevance.	
● Sleeping	Usually has difficulty in sleeping lying flat so uses 2 pillows. Otherwise sleeps well. Rises at 0530 hrs to start work.	● Breathlessness interfering with sleep.
● Dying		

- administration of oxygen
- activities to minimise oxygen requirement
- allaying anxiety

The rationale of these activities is explained below.

Maintaining patient in upright sitting position.
Lying flat, normally the most restful position, is contra-indicated when the patient is having difficulty in breathing because it further embarrasses breathing. When flat, the abdominal organs slide against the inferior aspect of the diaphragm and inhibit its movement, and the rib cage also has limited expansion. The lungs themselves have no muscles and are forced to expand and enabled to contract by the movement of the ribs (achieved by the intercostal muscles) and the diaphragm, a muscular partition between the thoracic and abdominal cavities.

Special beds may be available which help to maintain the upright sitting position. However when these are not available, as in Mr Morton's case, the patient can be maintained in this position well supported by pillows.

Administration of prescribed drugs. On admission, Mr Morton was given by the doctor, intravenously, a dose of aminophylline. This is a *bronchodilator*, a drug which, as the name suggests, dilates the bronchi and thus reduces the bronchospasm of asthma. Thereafter, Mr Morton was to be given another bronchodilator drug (salbutamol) every 4 hours by inhalation, using a nebuliser. The nebuliser provides a metered dose of 100 micrograms at each 'puff'; two puffs comprise one dose and maximum bronchodilation is achieved if the puffs are taken 5 minutes apart. Relief is usually obtained for three to four hours. As the nurse had already ascertained from Mrs Morton that the patient had been using this drug at home in recent weeks and knew how to use the nebuliser correctly, it was not necessary to disturb Mr Morton to explain the procedure.

To maximise the effect of the bronchodilator the doctor also administered by the intravenous route a dose of the hormone hydrocortisone, a *steroid* drug which has an anti-inflammatory and shrinking effect on the bronchial mucous membrane (which swells in an asthmatic attack). To prevent increase of anxiety in an already anxious patient, the nurse explained in simple terms the beneficial action of this drug.

The doctor then prescribed a course of the *steroid*, prednisolone, to be taken orally. This has a similar action to cortisone but with less side effect of salt and water retention. The goal to be achieved by this drug regime was to increase the volume of both inspired and expired air. This would be evaluated by daily estimations of the Forced Expiratory Volume (FEV) and the Forced Ventilatory Capacity (FVC) carried out by a technician. The nurse's responsibility would be to administer this drug as prescribed and explain its rationale to Mr Morton, and observe the effects.

Administration of oxygen. Mr Morton's laboured breathing together with his blue lips, cheeks and colour—observations made on admission—were evidence that his blood was deficient in oxygen. Objective assessment of whether or not the blood is adequately oxygenated is carried out by laboratory analysis of blood samples.

When there is prolonged reduction in the oxygen content of the patient's blood, the lack must be corrected by the addition of O_2 to the inhaled air. This was the reason given by the nurse to Mr Morton when oxygen therapy was commenced in response to the doctor's prescription. In Mr Morton's case, O_2 was administered by means of a nasal catheter (a 28 per cent concentration supplied at 2 litres per minute) as opposed to a mask, because it is less restricting and permits speech, eating and drinking without removal.

The nurse explained the wearing of the nasal catheter to Mr Morton, commenced the flow of oxygen and observed the necessary fire precautions. In order for the effectiveness of the O_2 therapy to be evaluated, goals must be set. These could be stated as:

- easier breathing
- red lips, pink cheeks/earlobes
- more relaxed patient

and evaluated by:

- counting respirations
- observing respirations; colour; affect
- asking patient how he feels
- (objectively, by blood gas measurements)

Activities to minimise oxygen requirement. Any exertion increases oxygen need and, when oxygen is in short supply, all possible ways of minimising O_2 requirement should be sought. Confining Mr Morton to bed is the first way of preventing him from unnecessary exertion and of promoting physical rest. However, a breathless person is often a distressed and very restless patient, and even sometimes panicky. The presence of a nurse, at least within sight, often helps the patient to feel less fearful and, as a result, to be more restful. For this reason, Mr Morton had been placed in a bed within direct vision of the nurses' observation point in the ward and he was shown how to use his call alarm and the buzzer was placed in his hand, ready to use.

Various other activities were carried out with the same goal of minimising Mr Morton's O_2 requirement. All procedures and events were explained to him before they occurred so that he did not have to ask unnecessary questions, thus minimising the need to speak which increases the effort required for breathing. When it was necessary to ask Mr Morton to speak, questions were phrased in such a way as to require the shortest possible answer.

When Mr Morton needed to move in bed, for example, to use a urinal, he was given assistance and encouraged to minimise the amount of movement. His locker was put close to the bed and in easy reach of his left hand (his preferred hand) to allow him easy access to his sputum carton, tumbler of water and his other possessions.

All nursing routines, apart from those which were absolutely necessary, were avoided during this critically ill phase. His priority problem was severe difficulty in breathing and only nursing interventions relevant to alleviating this problem were implemented in the first instance.

Allaying patient's anxiety. Activities and relatively minor anxieties with which he would normally cope, assume abnormal proportions when someone is fighting for breath. Initially, Mr Morton was extremely agitated and distressed and sought constant reassurance, first that he was not going to die, then that his wife would not go home and leave him and, later, that he would not be left by the nurse for even a minute. However, vigilance in explaining the nature of and reason for each intervention eventually achieved its goal: a less agitated and more relaxed patient.

NURSING INTERVENTION ONCE BREATHING IMPROVED

Within several hours, Mr Morton was breathing more easily, his colour had improved and he was relaxed and restful. The emergency treatment for his acutely ill condition had been effective.

At this stage it was appropriate to implement a further set of nursing activities, these being in relation to the AL of breathing and also to other ALs:

- teaching and supervising patient's breathing and coughing exercises
- attending to other ALs

Teaching patient breathing and coughing exercises. As soon as there was some improvement in Mr Morton's breathing, the physiotherapist visited him and taught him positional breathing exercises to move the accumulated sputum in order to maximise gaseous exchange between the air at the alveolar membrane and blood in the adjacent capillaries. An increased amount of thick secretions from the bronchioles is a feature of asthmatic attacks. The patient is instructed to breathe as deeply as possible to loosen the secretions and stimulate productive coughing. In order to cough effectively, the patient should breathe in deeply and breathe out with force. The nurse's responsibility is to reinforce the physiotherapist's instructions and encourage the patient to carry out the exercises regularly. At first Mr Morton was able to do the breathing and coughing exercises only when sitting up, but after a few days he was able to lie on his back, take a number of deep breaths, turn onto his side and expectorate. This was very effective and resulted in expectoration of copious sputum, followed by a gradual decline in the amount (as measured and recorded daily) and a corresponding improvement in his breathing.

Attending to other ALs. As the importance of maximum rest had been explained to Mr Morton, he was able to accept total dependence for his ALs during the period he was confined to bed. Examples of the nursing activities implemented in relation to the ALs concerned are given here, the goal of all being to minimise Mr Morton's requirement for oxygen:

AL	Nursing activities implemented	Goal
Eating and drinking	Semisolid diet, meals served in bed, drinks accessible on locker	
Eliminating	Urinal/bedpan as needed, assistance given onto bedpan, handwashing facilities provided	minimising Mr Morton's requirements for O_2
Personal cleansing and dressing	Bedbath; teeth cleaning facilities provided; assistance to comb hair/shave; assistance to alter position to relieve pressure	
Mobilising	Assistance given for all movement required; requirements placed within reach; call alarm provided	

Within 48 hours, once Mr Morton's breathing was no longer difficult while he was at rest, a gradual increase in his level of activity was encouraged. One of the first allowances was for Mr Morton to use a commode at his bedside and to assist with personal cleansing activities.

In order to attend to the patient's ALs in a personal way, data were obtained about his usual routines and habits— using basic facts from Mrs Morton when the Patient Assessment Form was first filled in and other details from the patient himself once he was sufficiently well to converse with the nurses. Data from the assessments of Mr Morton's ALs are entered on the right-hand side of his assessment form (Fig. 9.1).

NURSING INTERVENTION RELATED TO OTHER PROBLEMS

It can also be seen from these data concerning Mr Morton's ALs that this patient, in addition to those problems arising directly from his severe dyspnoea, has two other problems: excess weight and dental caries. Both are problems which Mr Morton himself could do something about and, during his recovery in hospital, he might be offered advice on these problems. His obesity could be tackled both in relation to his high carbohydrate intake (from food and beer) and his low exercise level. Dental caries could be explained to Mr Morton, preventive measures outlined and advice given to visit a dentist.

Considering other problems apparent in this patient serves to reinforce the idea that considering the relative priority of a patient's problems is a most important step in the process of nursing. On admission it was quite clear that Mr Morton had one life-threatening problem—severe dyspnoea. This had to be overcome before the other problems were considered. The ability to decide the priority of problems is an essential skill in using the process of nursing when nursing acutely ill patients.

10

Using the process when nursing a patient at home

The process of nursing can be applied in any situation—hospital or community. The kind of nursing intervention relevant in the two situations may be very different but the *process* remains the same.

Community nursing can involve for each patient/client/family, the phases of assessment, planning, implementation and evaluation. Community nursing is attractive to nurses who can only work part-time; some local authorities have a late evening shift, so for these and other reasons a written nursing plan is crucial so that the patient can receive 'planned' nursing. A written plan is also the means of rational long-term planning, intermittent evaluation and regular updating of goals. A clear statement of goals is very important in the community because much of their achievement depends on the patient himself; he therefore needs to be involved in setting realistic goals and evaluating his progress in relation to them.

As well as nursing sick people, community nurses—especially health visitors—play an important part in prevention of illness and promotion of health. The nursing process is relevant to this aspect of nursing too. For example, the health visitor with responsibility for pre-school children must carry out assessment of each child in order to identify potential problems, and set specific goals, before planning intervention. The intervention in this case is likely to be some form of health education which is as important a nursing activity as any of the more conventional nursing 'tasks'. In contrast, a health visitor's intermittent assessments of a frail old man living alone at home were presented in Chapter 3.

In some instances the problems of a patient/client in the community cannot be tackled by nurses alone. Some appropriate nursing activities therefore consist of referral to another professional group or organisation.

Cooperation between the district nurse and other health professionals is one aspect of the following study demonstrating use of the process of nursing in the community. The patient involved is Mr Elland, an elderly gentleman who suffered a stroke and whose rehabilitation is being continued at home.

MR FRANK ELLAND   Age 73
Recovering at home
from a stroke

At the age of 73 Mr Elland, a previously active and reasonably healthy man, while working in his garden was suddenly aware of weakness in his right side. He began to dribble saliva from his mouth, his vision was blurred and an attempt to call his wife did not produce intelligible words but merely grunts. He was conscious and consequently very frightened. His wife managed to get him into the house and immediately called the doctor who diagnosed a cerebrovascular accident (CVA). The doctor contacted the community nursing service and the district nurse visited later in the day, by which time a married daughter who lived nearby had arrived to lend her support.

ASSESSMENT ON REFERRAL

After an initial assessment of the environment and discussion with Mr and Mrs Elland and their daughter, it was decided that Mr Elland should stay in the double bed. There was enough space in the bedroom to place a commode at the bedside and the heating would allow Mr Elland to sit in a chair when able to do so. The room itself was situated next to a bathroom with toilet.

The district nurse, with Mrs Elland's assistance, helped make the patient comfortable, taking preventive measures against right-sided footdrop and wristdrop, and outlined for them his likely progress in the next few days. In the meantime she advised Mr Elland to rest until teatime. She

81

Patient Assessment Form

Date of ~~admission~~ *referral to District Nurse* 2 August

Date of assessment 2 August

Surname ELLAND

Forenames Frank

Male ☑

Female ☐

Age 73

Date of birth

~~Single~~/Married/~~Widowed~~ ✓

Other

Prefers to be addressed as

Mr Elland

Address of usual residence 12 Cedar Drive
Hillview Estate
Greenbank

Type of accommodation Detached bungalow with garden.

Family/~~Others~~ at this residence Wife

Next of kin Name Mrs Joan Elland Address as above

Relationship Wife Tel. no. Greenbank 473

Significant others Relatives/~~Dependents~~ 2 married daughters

Helpers Younger daughter who lives nearby

Visitors Family, friends, neighbours

Occupation Retired

Religious beliefs and relevant practices Church of England

Patient's perception of current health status Knows he has had a stroke.

Reason for ~~admission~~/referral Home nursing required / rehabilitation

Medical diagnosis C.V.A. R-sided hemiplegia

Past medical history Osteoarthritis (hips and lumbar spine). Hypertension reduced by loss of weight 5 years ago.

Allergies

Significant life crises

Fig. 10.1 Mr Elland: assessment with problems stated

Assessment of Activities of Living

Date 2 Aug.

AL	Usual routines: what he/she can and cannot do independently	Patient's problems (actual/potential) (p) = potential
● Maintaining a safe environment	Usually careful about safety; cautious due to age and limited mobility (osteoarthritis)	● Dependent
● Communicating	Intelligent. Large vocabulary, articulate before CVA. Now slurred speech, but able to recognise written and spoken word.	● Slurred speech
● Breathing	Breathes normally. Non-smoker.	
● Eating and drinking	Remains overweight, despite successful reduction 5 yrs ago. Can swallow food without difficulty since CVA but unable to feed self totally.	● Dependent for feeding ● Obesity
● Eliminating	Usually no problems. Continent of urine and faeces. Bowels regular (2-3 times per week).	● Dependent
● Personal cleansing and dressing	Usually bathes twice weekly, washes am and pm. Takes pride in appearance. Skin in good condition.	● Dependent ● (p) Pressure sores
● Controlling body temperature	Temperature within range of normal.	
● Mobilising	R-sided hemiplegia following CVA. Has had limited movement due to osteoarthritis. Can raise R arm above head; can straighten R knee when sitting in chair beside bed.	● Loss of ('aided') independence /R-sided hemiplegia
● Working and playing	Main interest/activity is gardening. Enjoys daily paper, cards, dominoes.	● Loss of mobilising for gardening
● Expressing sexuality	Nil of relevance.	
● Sleeping	Usually sleeps well (without medication) 2300 - 0700 hrs. Double bed; 2 pillows.	
● Dying		

then talked with Mrs Elland and her daughter and from them collected the biographical and health data on the left-hand side of the Patient Assessment Form (Fig. 10.1). The nurse explained about the articles required by her for attending to Mr Elland's personal toilet while he remained bedfast.

In the evening while carrying out Mr Elland's evening toilet, the nurse assessed his status on the dependence/independence continuum for several ALs and Mrs Elland supplied some of the data recorded on the right side of the form.

IDENTIFYING MR ELLAND'S PROBLEMS

Analysis of the assessment data showed that several of Mr Elland's problems stemmed from his loss of independence for mobilising because it inter-related with several other ALs. But in fact it was loss of *aided* independence because he had previously used a walking stick to take some of his weight in order to protect his osteoarthritic hips and lumbar spine. Several other problems were identified:

- loss of 'aided' independence for mobilising, including
  personal grooming and cleanliness
  dressing
  eliminating
  (gardening: Mr Elland's main hobby)

- potential: pressure sores
- obesity
- dependence for feeding
- slurred speech

PLANNING INTERVENTION RELEVANT TO THESE PROBLEMS

Since Mr and Mrs Elland would be closely concerned with carrying out the interventions to achieve the goals set, it was imperative that they cooperated in, and understood that a record would be kept of goal achievement. Some long- and some short-term goals were set and they understood the importance of recording the smaller day-to-day improvement in Mr Elland's ability to carry out even simple tasks.

Problem: loss of 'aided' independence for mobilising

The psychological trauma resulting from this sort of loss, can be likened to that inflicted by loss of a limb or a breast, or to that experienced in bereavement, and the necessary nursing intervention is included in Mr Elland's nursing plan:

Problem	Goal	Nursing intervention	Evaluation
Psychological trauma	Positive feeling towards rehabilitation	Encourage frank discussion of their reaction to their predicament	Cooperating in rehabilitation

To achieve the two goals of adequate movement in the right lower limb and prevention of deformity, the nursing intervention was to teach appropriate exercises to be carried out at first in bed. The community physiotherapist had worked these out in conjunction with the nurses. After

a week the doctor arranged additional rehabilitation at the nearby day hospital which Mr Elland attended twice weekly for three months. The long-term goals were written on the nursing plan:

Problem	Goal	Nursing intervention	Evaluation
Loss of 'aided' independence for mobilising	Adequate movement in R. upper and lower limbs Absence of deformity Stand/walk with tall/short frame	Teach/supervise: bed exercises transfer skills Standing/walking with tall/short walking frame	

Name	Date	Physical Condition A Good 4 Fair 3 Poor 2 V. bad 1	Mental condition B Alert 4 Apathetic 3 Confused 2 Stuporous 1	Activity C Ambulant 4 Walk/help 3 Chairbound 2 Bedfast 1	Mobility D Full 4 Sl. limited 3 V. limited 2 Immobile 1	Incontinent E Not 4 Occasionally 3 Usually/ur. 2 Doubly 1	Total score

Fig. 10.2 Norton scoring scale

Loss of sensation in the right side gave rise to a postural problem when standing. In view of Mr Elland's height and weight, a tall walking frame was acquired; it not only gave a wide base support but also provided support on all sides and therefore lessened fear of falling. When sufficient strength and confidence were gained the goal changed to walking with a lower frame. This goal was achieved three months later when he was discharged from twice weekly attendance at the day hospital.

However improvement can be expected up to two years after a CVA; it is possible that he may achieve further independence and may come to prefer using a tripod walking stick/cane or even a simple stick/cane. His level of independence for, and style of mobilising when he was discharged from the day hospital is, therefore, not the end of the story: his further progress will be carefully monitored and recorded each month by the district nurse.

To achieve the goal of adequate movement in the upper limb, necessary for carrying out so many activities, the nursing intervention was to teach appropriate exercises— again with advice from the physiotherapist when necessary. Mr Elland agreed to use his right hand and arm as much as he possibly could. Mr and Mrs Elland were both interested in and agreed to keep a detailed record of Mr Elland's daily achievement in his everyday living activities involving the right upper limb, so that progress could be monitored by the district nurse.

Potential problem: pressure sores
Pressure sore risk assessment was carried out using the Norton scoring system (Fig. 10.2). Patients with a total score of 14 or less are liable to develop pressure sores and when the score is lower than 12 the risk is very high.

Because Mr Elland was obese and there was a sensory impairment on the right side his A score was 1; B was 4; C was 1; since he could not move the right side of his body and in view of the restricted movement in his left hip and lumbar spine, the D score was 2, and the E score 4, making a total of 12. The nursing intervention to prevent this potential problem becoming an actual one was teaching Mr and Mrs Elland about regular relief of pressure over the bony prominences. Early acquisition of transfer skills helped, and Mr Elland understood that rising from the chair for even half a minute would relieve pressure and he was willing to do this. A full length sheepskin over the bottom sheet of the bed prevented damage during the night.

Problem: obesity
Mr Elland was aware of this problem and was concerned that he was so heavy for his relatives and the nurses to lift and support. He was 1.8 m (5ft 10in) in height and weighed 95 kg (15 stone); he was of large body frame, so taking all these factors into consideration, a desirable weight would be 72–81 kg. It was decided by all concerned that a realistic goal would be loss of 6 kg in each month. To accomplish this, and taking food and fluid likes and dislikes into consideration, a daily diet of approximately 4200 kilojoules (1000 Calories) was planned. To give Mr Elland practice in improving his diminished writing skills he laboriously made out a weight graph and took great pleasure in recording the downward slope on it, confirming that the goal was being achieved.

What was written on the nursing plan in relation to Mr Elland's obesity problem is shown below:

Problem	Goal	Nursing intervention	Evaluation	(Date)
Overweight	Loss of weight from 95 to 72–81 kg	Teach good eating habits	95kg	9/8
		Supervise 4200 kJ diet	89kg	9/9
		Praise weight loss	86kg	9/10
			82kg	9/11

Tackling an overweight problem is never easy and at 73 Mr Elland might well have asked 'Is it worth it?' As a previously active man, increased independence in mobilising was very important to him, so the interrelatedness of the ALs played a part in motivating him to lose weight. Consideration for those who would have to lift him, should he be ill again, also motivated him.

Problem: dependence for feeding
During the first week Mr Elland was fed with semisolids by his wife. Although towards the end of the second week he could feed himself slowly and with minimal spillage using the left hand, he remained dependent on his wife for cutting solid food. At the end of a month's attendance at the day hospital the occupational therapist procured a piece of cutlery which acts as an all-in-one knife, fork and spoon. This permitted cutting of solid food with the left hand and thus feeding ceased to be a problem and the nursing plan was updated:

Problem	Goal	Nursing intervention	Evaluation
2/8 Dependent for eating	Independent feeding with L hand	Semisolid food	
		Introduce solid food	
			16/8 Dependent cutting solid food, independent slow feeding with L hand, minimal spillage
		2/9 Occupational therapist all-in-one cutlery	
			5/9 'Aided' independence, problem solved

However, it is hoped that with use of the muscles of the right forearm for several other ALs they will become sufficiently strong to permit resumption of use of a knife and fork.

Problem: slurred speech

Speech problems are common after a cerebrovascular accident. For the majority of people speech is the most commonly used medium for communicating with others, so any impediment is problematic. Fortunately for Mr Elland his aphasia was of the expressive type, i.e., although he had difficulty in articulating words because the lesion was in the motor speech area, he retained the ability to recognise both the spoken and written word. Weakness in the many muscles required for speaking caused his speech to be markedly slurred and disfigured his face. In dealing with these problems he had therefore to learn to cope with feelings of embarrassment and frustration.

Discussion between the nurse and the speech therapist resulted in formulation of a nursing plan which instructed nurses to encourage his performance of specific lip and tongue exercises six times daily. He found it easier to remember the times as before and after breakfast, lunch and supper. In addition, speaking practice was to be encouraged. As Mr Elland was an inveterate newspaper reader he agreed to read a portion aloud to his wife morning and evening. Mrs Elland was asked to encourage her husband to talk throughout the day. A further source of practice was conversation with his daughters and their children and other visitors.

At the end of two weeks' attendance at the day hospital, the speech therapist's evaluation stated that Mr Elland's face was now normal but he was speaking too quickly and became confused over long sentences. He was advised and constantly encouraged to speak more slowly. Gradually he became more confident and increasingly more competent at speaking. At the end of three months, when he was discharged from the day hospital, regular exercises and practice were no longer necessary as it was only when Mr Elland was tired or upset that a slight impediment could be detected, as summarised on the nursing plan:

Problem	Goal	Nursing intervention	Evaluation
2/8 Slurred speech	Speaking intelligibly	Encourage lip and tongue exercises × 6 daily Read aloud M and E Encourage speaking practice	
		Encourage slower speaking	*23/8* Face normal Speaking too quickly, confused over long sentences
			9/11 Slight impediment only when tired or upset

This chapter shows how members of a multidisciplinary team made their contribution while a patient received home care followed by attendance at a day hospital. Supervision and encouragement or reinforcement of all Mr Elland's activities was the district nurse's responsibility throughout. Most important, the usefulness to all concerned of an organised, documented nursing plan in process format which helped Mr Elland's achievement of his goal—coping adequately at home—has been demonstrated.

11

Using the process in preoperative nursing

Any patient who consents to have an operation entrusts his faith in the skill and care of the surgical team. Nobody likes the idea of surgery. Some people are terror-stricken at the prospect. And it is a fact that surgery carries serious risks to life and safety. So, for all of these reasons, nursing a patient who is about to have an operation is a very serious and challenging responsibility.

Increasingly, it is being realised that psychological preparation for surgery is an important nursing function. The research studies of Hayward (1975) and Boore (1978), showing the value of preoperative information giving, have done much to make nurses aware of the importance of this aspect of preoperative nursing.

Two aspects of preoperative nursing will be considered here: firstly, the ways in which data collected from assessment of ALs on admission influence the patient's nursing; secondly, 'routine' preoperative measures are considered in relation to ALs.

The patient is Mrs Murray, a young woman admitted for cholecystectomy.

MRS PATRICIA MURRAY   Age 35

Admitted for cholecystectomy

Over a period of 4 months Mrs Murray had been troubled by pain in the right hypochondrium. The pain consisted of a dull ache practically all of the time, with bouts of quite excruciating pain which radiated into her back. The onset of this more severe pain did not seem to be related to food—even to fatty foods—but Mrs Murray also complained of heartburn and, sometimes, water-brash and flatulence. Suspecting that this patient may be suffering from gall-

stones (cholelithiasis), the GP arranged with the hospital for Mrs Murray to have a cholecystogram (a particular X-ray investigation which demonstrates gall-bladder appearance and function). This, in fact, showed that the gall-bladder contained at least one large stone and it was recommended that Mrs Murray's name should be put on the waiting list for admission to hospital for cholecystectomy (removal of gall-bladder).

ASSESSMENT ON ADMISSION

On admission to the surgical ward on 20th July, for the operation planned to take place two days later, Mrs Murray was carefully assessed by the nurse and the ward doctor (the surgeon and the anaesthetist would visit the following day to introduce themselves to Mrs Murray, check that she was fit to undergo surgery as planned, and prescribe any special preoperative preparation and a premedication).

Information collected in the course of the nursing assessment is presented on the Patient Assessment Form (see Fig. 11.1). On the left-hand side of the form is the relevant biographical and health data. Immediately, it is clear that Mrs Murray's family/domestic circumstances are relevant to planning her nursing.

She has a young son, and because her husband works night shift, her mother-in-law has moved into the home to look after the child while Mrs Murray is in hospital. The patient is bound to be anxious about the child's welfare and Mr Murray will be unable to visit at the official visiting times.

Indeed, as can be seen in the list of patient's problems on the right side of the Patient Assessment Form, Mrs Murray's enforced separation from her husband and son is the specific cause of the problems identified in relation to the ALs of maintaining a safe environment and working and playing. Some problems listed are actual problems: those present on admission (e.g., constipation) or as a direct result of admission to hospital for a cholecystectomy (e.g., deprived of usual work activities/changed sleeping pattern).

It is not difficult to appreciate that the presence of these problems has implications for both pre- and postoperative nursing. Take, for example, the problem of constipation. If Mrs Murray has not achieved prevention of constipation immediately prior to admission, her rectum may contain an excess of hardening faeces. This, after a day or two of enforced bed rest following the operation, will result in an uncomfortable level of constipation in the postoperative period. It may delay or make difficult the first bowel evacuation and will almost certainly cause the patient a good deal of consternation. Therefore, it would be wise to use an enema preoperatively to empty the lower part of the gastrointestinal tract and, postoperatively to instruct Mrs Murray how she can use position and muscles to assist with defaecation and later to ensure that she receives a diet high in fibre-containing foods.

In a similar way, each of the problems identified from the admission assessment would be considered and relevant nursing activities planned for both the pre- and postoperative period. Thus, it can be seen that data collected from assessment on admission greatly influence the patient's nursing.

A summary of the kinds of nursing activities relevant in the preoperative nursing plan in relation to these problems identified from the assessment data follows:

AL	Problem	Intervention
Maintaining a safe environment	1. Unable to continue role in ensuring safety of child	Encourage mother-in-law to phone and visit with the child to reassure patient.
Communicating	2. Anxiety about specific aspects of surgery	Establish rapport with/confidence in staff. Explain the forthcoming operation, including preoperative preparation and postoperative management. Answer specific questions. Teach specific procedures which will contribute to postoperative recovery (including deep breathing and leg exercises).
Eating and drinking	3. Gastrointestinal discomforts	Advise patient to avoid foods which appear to be related to indigestion and flatulence.
	4. Overweight	Discuss with patient possibility of commencing reducing diet prior to discharge.
Eliminating	5. Constipation	Prevent undue anxiety about this problem. Administer enema on evening before operation. Discuss postoperative management with patient.
	6. Piles	Plan to prevent constipation postoperatively and teach patient prior to discharge methods of preventing constipation. Local application of analgesic, if necessary.
Mobilising	7. Habitual lack of exercise	Discuss importance of cooperating in postoperative exercise regime. Teach deep breathing and leg exercises.
Working and playing	8. Deprived of usual work and parental roles	Help patient to plan activities during preoperative period in order to prevent boredom and avoid undue anxiety and distress at separation from child. Encourage her to have family visitors.
	9. Husband unable to visit at official visiting times	Discuss possible alternative visiting regime and make arrangements to accommodate this. Arrange for bedside phone to be available postoperatively.
Sleeping	10. Changed sleeping pattern in hospital	Encourage relaxation prior to bedtime on the 2 preoperative nights. Ask doctor to prescribe sleeping tablets if necessary.

Patient Assessment Form

Date of admission *20 July*   Date of assessment *20 July*

Surname *MURRAY*   Forenames *Patricia*

Male ☐   Age ☐ *35*   ~~Single~~/Married ✓/~~Widowed~~   Prefers to be addressed as
Female ☑   Other   *Mrs Murray*

Date of birth

Address of usual residence *127 East Mains Avenue, Newtown*

Type of accommodation *Terraced 2-bedroom house (rented), with bathroom*

Family/~~Others~~ at this residence *Husband and son (age 7) (Mother-in-law staying while Mrs M is in hospital)*

Next of kin   Name *Mr Tom Murray*   Address *as above*

          Relationship *Husband*   Tel. no. {*063-7243 at work: 063-8181 ext 212*

Significant others   Relatives/Dependents *Husband and son*

          Helpers *Mother-in-law*

          Visitors *Family as above*

Occupation *Part-time typist / housewife*

Religious beliefs and relevant practices *None*

Patient's perception of current health status *Understands she is to have her gall bladder removed and expects this to cure her problems.*

Reason for admission/~~referral~~ *Cholecystectomy*

Medical diagnosis *Cholelithiasis*

Past medical history *Piles causing intermittent rectal bleeding for 18/12 following birth o[...]*

Allergies *None*   Significant life crises *None recent*

Fig. 11.1 Mrs Murray: assessment with problems stated

Assessment of Activities of Living

Date *20 July*

AL	Usual routines: what he/she can and cannot do independently	Patient's problems (actual/potential) (p) = potential
● Maintaining a safe environment	Expresses anxiety about safety of home and family, especially child, in her absence in hospital.	● Deprived of role in ensuring safety of child
● Communicating	Communicates with ease. Evidence of anxiety about operation, in particular concerning pain afterwards.	● Anxiety about aspects of surgery.
● Breathing	Non-smoker. No breathing problems. Does not have a cold or cough. Respirations 16/min.	
● Eating and drinking	Appetite unaffected by pain and other discomforts (waterbrash, heartburn, flatulence), although has cut down on fat intake. Overweight for height	● Gastrointestinal discomforts ● Overweight
● Eliminating	Suffers from chronic constipation and very painful piles. Likes to defaecate daily and takes bran to achieve this. No problems with micturition.	● Constipation ● Piles
● Personal cleansing and dressing	Twice weekly bath/hairwash. Has full dentures.	
● Controlling body temperature	Temperature on admission 36°c.	
● Mobilising	Fully mobile, but takes little exercise and feels rather unfit most of the time.	● Habitual lack of exercise
● Working and playing	Leads a busy life as part-time typist and housewife/mother. Husband works night-shift. Has no hobbies, only leisure pursuit is TV.	● Deprived of usual work and parental roles ● Husband unable to visit at official visiting times
● Expressing sexuality	Last menstrual period finished 14/7. Is not on contraceptive pill.	
● Sleeping	Usually sleeps well 2330-0630 hrs. Prefers duvet and no pillow. Anxious that she will not be able to sleep in hospital.	● Changed sleeping pattern in hospital
● Dying		

'ROUTINE' PREOPERATIVE MEASURES

In addition to the interventions already suggested above, a further set of nursing activities has to be planned to prepare the patient for surgery. It is also possible to consider these 'routine' preoperative measures in relation to relevant ALs.

AL	Nursing activities involved in preparation of patient for cholecystectomy
Maintaining a safe environment	Plan preparation of bed and bed area for safe postoperative nursing. Consider possible safety hazards in her postoperative period and plan to minimise risks. Reassure patient that her personal safety is being considered.
Communicating	Psychological preparation for surgery (explanation, teaching, establishing rapport, alleviating anxiety) in order to assist successful postoperative recovery.
Breathing	Record preoperative TPR and BP Teach deep breathing exercises and explain importance of preventing respiratory complications postoperatively.
Eating and drinking	Nil by mouth regime to start 6–8 hours preoperatively,[1] Mrs Murray for theatre at 0800 hours so fast from midnight (offer patient tea and biscuits as near to that time as she wishes). Nasogastric tube to be passed prior to transfer to theatre. This permits stomach to be as empty as possible, thus minimising the risk of aspiration of vomit while under anaesthetic and recovering from anaesthesia. Procedure to be explained to Mrs Murray.
Eliminating	Enema on night before operation. Enable Mrs Murray to empty bladder as soon as possible before transfer to theatre.
Personal cleansing and dressing	Immersion bath on morning of operation (this minimises the micro-organic count of the skin). Shave entire abdomen from costal margins as far as and including the pubis, using a sharp razor and shave against the grain, avoiding cutting skin.[2] Dress in theatre gown (and, if used, hat/socks) and remove dentures and jewellery (and if relevant prosthesis, contact lenses, hair pins); strap wedding ring and attach personal identity band to wrist or ankle.
Controlling body temperature	Preoperative temperature to be recorded on TPR chart. Ensure patient is comfortably warm once dressed for theatre.
Mobilising	Teach leg exercises to assist in prevention of DVT postoperatively. Explain the graduated mobilising routine postoperatively and stress the importance of body movement.
Sleeping	Promote maximum rest and relaxation. Administer prescribed sleeping tablets if needed.

[1] Hamilton-Smith (1972) from a study of preoperative fasting urges times of fasting to be considered on an individual basis rather than as a routine nursing practice.

[2] There is some evidence that depilatory creams result in a lower micro-organic count (Powis et al, 1976).

In addition to the above nursing measures, the patient undergoes medical preparation prior to surgery. For Mrs Murray this would include:

- correction of any nutritional deficiencies
- correction of any fluid and electrolyte imbalance
- ensuring adequate blood volume
- checking the prothrombin index (this is always done prior to cholecystectomy, particularly if the patient has had biliary obstruction which has prevented the absorption of vitamin K)
- management of any acute/chronic infection
- obtaining consent of patient for operation
- prescribing premedication

Even this fairly brief description of the various activities involved in preoperative nursing serves to show how complex it is. Not only is there the 'routine' preparation of the patient for surgery, but also essential is attention to the individual patient's problems, as identified from assessment on admission. The model for nursing with its focus on ALs, provides a useful framework for both of these aspects of pre-operative nursing, as illustrated in relation to Mrs Murray.

REFERENCES

Boore J 1978 Prescription for recovery. Royal College of Nursing, London
Hamilton Smith S 1972 Nil by mouth. Royal College of Nursing, London
Hayward J 1975 Information—a prescription against pain. Royal College of Nursing, London
Powis S, Waterworth T, Arkell D 1976 Preoperative skin preparation: clinical evaluation of depilatory cream. British Medical Journal 2: 1166–1168

12

Using the process in postoperative nursing

For experienced surgical nurses, postoperative nursing becomes a familiar routine which is carried out efficiently and with confidence. The observer of the practised nurse's skill, speed and calm approach cannot but be impressed, and, at the same time, bewildered by the apparent complexity and tremendous responsibility of the nurse's task. The inexperienced nursing student, or the mature nurse resuming her career after a break, is likely to feel just the same as the observer, on watching their senior colleague operate with such alacrity.

One of the very valuable uses of the nursing process is that it provides a structured framework for the breakdown of highly complex nursing activities. Thus, the various separate actions in a complex nursing activity can be identified, the rationale for their implementation can be clarified and related to the underlying data (from assessment); goals of nursing can be specified and the method of evaluation detailed. All of this information, in great or minimal detail, can be included in a patient's nursing plan.

For the experienced nurse, a written plan may seem almost unnecessary. She is able to amass all the data in her head and, repeating the process of nursing with amazing rapidity, achieve the goals set. However, for the learner, a detailed nursing plan can be her guide and, if it contains explanation of the rationale of the interventions planned, it can also be her teacher. An example of a detailed written plan is presented below. It concerns the immediate postoperative nursing of Mrs Murray, the patient discussed in Chapter 11. Her Patient Assessment Form can be found in Figure 11.1 on page 90.

TABLE 12.1 MRS MURRAY: POSTOPERATIVE NURSING PLAN

Goal	Potential problem	Reason for problem	Related assessment
Maintaining adequate ventilation	Acute respiratory obstruction	Loss of swallowing reflex and control of jaw musculature under anaesthesia	Check tongue is not occluding airway
		When recovering from anaesthetic tongue may fall back and obstruct airway	Observe breathing and note signs of O_2 insufficiency increased rate shallow noise cyanosis rapid weak pulse restlessness
		Inhalation of vomit/mucus	

MRS PATRICIA MURRAY   Age 35

Recovering from cholecystectomy

Mrs Murray had her operation on 22 July. Her gall-bladder showed typical signs of chronic inflammation, being thick-walled and scarred; two large gallstones were removed from it. Sometimes after the gall-bladder has been taken out, the common bile duct may then be explored for further stones: this was done in Mrs Murray's case. As this exploration can result in oedema, it is necessary for a T-tube drain to be inserted to allow free flow of bile from the liver. A drainage tube is always inserted into the gall-bladder bed at the end of the operation to drain accumulated fluid and prevent the formation of a haematoma. This drain is brought out through the wound or through a separate stab wound according to the surgeon's preference. The wound is closed and a dressing applied. Mrs Murray's operation was completed without any complications.

In readiness for the patient's return, the bed and bed area had been prepared. Such preparation is an important part of the planning phase of the nursing process, involving as it does consideration of the physical environment and availability of equipment and personnel (pp 4–5).

For Mrs Murray's return the following equipment was in readiness:

- airway
- sphygmomanometer and stethoscope
- intravenous infusion stand
- equipment for oxygen therapy
- suction apparatus
- equipment for nasogastric aspiration
- disposable oral hygiene packs

At 11.30 hours the ward received a telephone call from the recovery room to say that Mrs Murray was ready for transfer to the ward. The ward nurse was given the postoperative note and orders written by the doctor.

- BP 100/70 : pulse 100 per minute
  Recordings to be made $\frac{1}{2}$ hourly
- 2 drains in situ:
  1 ragnal drain in gall-bladder bed
  1 T-tube drain in bile duct
  attached to free drainage
- IVI in progress, 500 ml Dextrose 5 % (to be through by 13.00, followed by 500 ml normal saline in 4 hours, thereafter alternating 4 hourly; fluid balance chart to be maintained)
- to be given nil by mouth
- analgesia (Omnopon 15 mg i.m.) to be given 4 hourly first dose due at 15.00 hours (diamorphine 5 mg given at 11.00)

POSTOPERATIVE NURSING PLAN

The immediate postoperative period is a crucial one and the nurse plays a major part in the overall objectives, namely:

- to ensure the patient's complete recovery from anaesthesia
- to prevent the onset of postoperative complications

Within these overall objectives the following major nursing goals are considered in the postoperative nursing plan presented in tabular form below:

- maintaining adequate ventilation
- preventing shock
- preventing chest infection
- preventing venous stasis
- effectively alleviating pain
- preventing urinary infection

Relevant interventions	Rationale for intervention	Goals for evaluation
Use left lateral position	To help to prevent tongue from falling back or vomit being inhaled	Steady, unlaboured, quiet breathing
Aspirate N/G tube hourly	To remove secretions in stomach	Pulse not unduly rapid (i.e., not more than 110 per min)
Encourage patient to cough up sputum	To remove excess sputum from respiratory tract	Satisfactory colour (i.e., not cyanosed)
Take immediate action if airway becomes obstructed
pull jaw forward and insert artificial airway
call the doctor	Oxygen deprivation results in brain damage, eventually death	

Evaluation:
Mrs Murray's pulse was 100/min and respirations 12/min on return from theatre and, within 1 hour stabilised at pulse 70–90/min resp 14–16/min. She showed no signs of respiratory distress, had complete control over tongue and coughing. Recordings taken hourly after 4 hours, continued to be satisfactory.

TABLE 12.1 Continued

Goal	Potential problem	Reason for problem	Related assessment
Preventing shock	Shock	May be due to failure of the heart to act as an effective pump or more commonly, the result of decreased volume of circulating blood being returned to the heart. The latter could occur from haemorrhage, severe fluid loss.	Observe for signs of shock: rapid thready pulse fall in BP pallor cyanotic lips cold moist skin fall in body temperature restlessness Check wound (front and back) for signs of haemorrhage Check drains are functioning and for signs of excessive fluid/blood loss
Preventing chest infection	Pneumonia	Susceptibility to chest infection because of: anaesthetic agents endotracheal tubes depression of ability to cough and expectorate aspiration of vomit/mucus prolonged immobility on operating table and in postoperative period which may decrease chest expansion. (Susceptibility increased in obese patients and smokers.)	Observe for signs of chest infection: increased body temperature cough infected sputum chest pain
Preventing venous stasis	Deep venous thrombosis of the calf vessels	Although the problem does not usually manifest until a week or so after surgery, causes include: compression of femoral or popliteal veins if the patient's knees are kept flexed for long periods increased viscosity of the blood postoperatively which causes increased coagulability and may result in DVT venous stasis due to immobility in the postoperative period	Check that leg veins are not being constricted Check skin temperature of each calf and body temperature Check for pain and tenderness in each calf

Relevant interventions	Rationale for intervention	Goals for evaluation
Move patient carefully	Minimise disturbance to wound and drains which could dislodge ligature	No sign of shock Stable BP and pulse
Adhere to prescribed i.v. fluid input	To maintain fluid volume and electrolyte balance	No sign of blood or fluid loss
Report to doctor signs of shock	Early diagnosis of cause and commencement of treatment is essential	(because haemorrhage may not become apparent for several hours regular evaluation is necessary throughout the first 24 hours

Evaluation:
Mrs Murray's BP, pulse, wound and drains were checked $\frac{1}{2}$ hourly for 4 hours. Her BP on admission was 120/80 and postoperatively it dropped to 100/70 2 hours after return from theatre, but thereafter stabilised at 110/70. Pulse was satisfactory at 70-90/min. No leakage was observed from the wound; no excess fluid escaped from either drain although both drains were functioning. Mrs Murray did not suffer from shock in the first 24 hours postoperatively.

Protect patient from sources of infection (other patients/staff with coughs and colds)	Avoids pathogenic microorganisms	No sign of chest infection:
		  normal body temperature
		  no cough
		  sputum clear
		  no chest pain

Encourage patient to sit up and perform deep breathing at intervals	Allows maximum chest expansion	
Encourage/help patient to cough at regular intervals (e.g., at each hourly recording session) and expectorate excess secretions	Removes excess secretions	
Implement schedule of gradual rehabilitation	Assists restoration of respiratory function	
Cooperate with physiotherapist		

Evaluation:
Mrs Murray had no preoperative problems with breathing and is a non-smoker, therefore less likely to develop problems postoperatively. She was able to sit up and cough 4 hours after her operation and quickly mastered the art of deep breathing and coughing. Her temperature, taken 4 hourly for the first 24 hours, remained at its pre-operative level, approx. 36°C.

Encourage patient to move legs in bed, especially flexion and extension of the knees and dorsiflexion of the ankles	Muscle action encourages venous flow/prevents stasis	Preventive measures being observed No signs or symptoms of DVT
Position patient correctly avoiding crossing of the legs	Prevents compression of veins	
Use/check elastic stockings if prescribed	Assists venous return	
Encourage early remobilisation	Promotes venous return	

Evaluation:
Mrs Murray carried out leg exercises when prompted at times when vital signs were being recorded. She was helped to sit out of bed for $\frac{1}{2}$ hour during bedmaking in the morning (i.e., almost 24 hours following operation). No warning signs of DVT were apparent in the immediate postoperative period.

TABLE 12.1 Continued

Goal	Potential problem	Reason for problem	Related assessment
Effectively alleviating pain	Undesirable consequences of pain: fatigue anxiety restlessness discomfort	Pain is an unpleasant sensation and may interfere with sleep and relaxation and cause anxiety and distress. Biliary surgery is known to be among the most painful surgical procedures (Bond, 1979)	Observe for signs of pain, e.g., restlessness Evaluate: locality severity temporal pattern relationship to e.g., movement Ask patient to describe pain using 'painometer' (Fig. 12.1)
Preventing urinary infection	Retention causing: discomfort from distended bladder restlessness stasis of urine resulting in infection	Pathogenic microorganisms have time to multiply excessively Bladder when full protrudes into abdominal cavity	Urine output Signs of bladder distension Discomfort

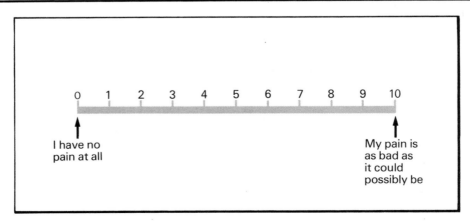

Fig. 12.1 Painometer

Relevant interventions	Rationale for intervention	Goals for evaluation
Administer analgesics regularly as prescribed	Regular administration keeps pain constantly under control	Patient comfortable and relaxed/sleeping
Maintain patient in comfortable position, avoid tension on wound and drains, carry out nursing procedures when pain control is at its optimum	Movement increases pain	Patient says there is no pain (painometer, see Fig. 12.1)
		Analgesics administered regularly as prescribed
Allow patient time and opportunity to discuss pain experienced/anticipated	Pain likely to be less well tolerated if patient anxious	

Evaluation:

Mrs Murray woke at 14.00 hours, 3 hours following operation and said she was in 'absolute agony'. Repositioning did not relieve the pain and she quickly became restless and noisy. The doctor confirmed that the first dose of Omnopon could be given. After the injection Mrs Murray quickly went to sleep and throughout the rest of the day and the first night the analgesic regime and careful positioning kept the patient relatively free of pain. Mrs Murray was prescribed Omnopon 15 mg (i.m.) 4 hourly. She was given a dose at 14.00, 17.00, 21.00, 01.10, 05.15 and 09.05 hours. The morning dose was given around 09.00 hours; bedmaking and physiotherapy were scheduled to follow at 10.00 hours when pain control would be at its maximum.

Assist patient to use bedpan/urinal	May stimulate micturition	No sign of discomfort from bladder distension
Report failure to void within 8–10 hours postoperatively	Retention possible within this time	No signs of urinary tract infection
Catheterise patient, if instructed	To remove urine from bladder in first instance, then to drain bladder	Patient voids within 8 to 10 hours
Catheter hygiene		Fluid input and output in balance

Evaluation:

Mrs Murray was helped to sit on a bedpan at 16.00 hours, 7 hours after return from theatre, but she was unable to pass urine. At 22.30 she complained of wanting to pass urine but not feeling able to and, on medical advice, she was catheterised. 200 ml of urine were obtained. By 06.00 the following morning, urine output totalled 2000 ml, an amount in balance with input.

The preceding nursing plan outlines the major goals of the immediate postoperative period and, it is clear, that nursing plays a most important role in ensuring the patient's complete recovery from anaesthesia and in preventing the onset of postoperative complications. Mrs Murray's progress in the period immediately following the cholecystectomy was fairly uneventful. She did experience severe pain for a short time in the early hours following the operation, but afterwards pain was well controlled. In addition she had to be catheterised because she did not manage to empty her bladder within the first 8 to 10 hours.

There are many different crucial nursing activities involved in immediate postoperative nursing. The usefulness of detailing them on a written nursing plan is to remind nurses of the necessary interventions and most important, to point out that the majority of these are aimed at preventing potential problems becoming actual ones, rather than management of actual problems. This is a point which emerges very clearly from the selected aspects of the postoperative nursing plan documented in this section.

REFERENCE

Bond M R 1979 Pain: its nature, analysis and treatment. Churchill Livingstone, Edinburgh, p 161

13

Using the process in patient teaching

It is not usual, even where written nursing plans are in use, to find nurses making plans for patient teaching and writing down these plans. In fact, few nurses seem to appreciate the necessity of *planning* teaching at all.

All good teachers plan their teaching. Many readers will be able to recall their teachers of years past entering the classroom and announcing with great purpose: 'Today, we are going to . . .'. That teacher was outlining the lesson plan which would have been part of an overall plan, prepared with objectives in mind and an evaluation system built in.

A nurse's teaching role is not envisaged as such a formal business—indeed, informality is more appropriate as a rule—but, nevertheless the analogy with the professional teacher is useful in reinforcing the idea that, to be effective, teaching must be planned. At present, much of the teaching done by nurses is carried out on an ad hoc basis, often only in direct response to a request for information from a patient. This means that patients, who are too anxious or lacking in knowledge, may not ask and, therefore, will not be given essential information. Or else, the well-meaning nurse will bombard the patient with information, about everything from drugs to exercise regulation, just as he is packing to go home from hospital with the inevitable result that information is confused or forgotten. Sometimes nurses rely on pamphlets for information without assessing whether or not the patients in question have the ability to comprehend them.

Many new skills will have to be acquired by nurses as patient teaching becomes an increasingly important part of their function.

The following presentation illustrates the planning of a teaching programme for a patient recovering from a myocardial infarction.

MR HENRY WOLF   Age 54
Learning to modify ALs
after a myocardial infarction

On May 8th, Henry Wolf, a 54-year-old schoolteacher, had a myocardial infarction. He was admitted to the coronary care unit of the nearby general hospital and a week later, having made excellent progress, was moved to a general medical ward. There within a day or two he was considered well enough to begin to take short walks—e.g., to the toilet—and gradually to increase independence in the ALs. Realising that his condition was improving daily and that he had escaped the major complications following myocardial infarction, Mr Wolf began to consider the future and the possible changes in his life which might now be necessary. It is inevitable that, following infarction, a patient and his family will feel anxious and uncertain about the future, so nurses have the challenging job of helping such patients to understand their position and, if necessary, to permanently modify their life-style to ensure recovery and to minimise the risk of a recurrence.

The fact that Mr Wolf, almost 2 weeks after suffering a myocardial infarction, was beginning to ask questions and express anxiety about his future, indicated that he was ready to be given more information and discuss his various worries with the staff. At this point the ward sister explained to him that it was her policy to discuss with patients who had had a myocardial infarction the topic of smoking (not applicable in his case), exercise, rest and diet and, if wished, sexual activity. She asked if there were other subjects he wanted to know about. Mr Wolf was pleased that he was to have the opportunity to be given information about these topics. He asked if, in addition, his doctor would go over, once more, the medical aspects of his condition and tell him whether or not he would be required to take any drugs on a long-term basis. Sister agreed to arrange a session with the doctor. Finally, she asked Mr Wolf whether he would like to involve his wife in their discussion and he agreed this would be desirable.

In order for Mr Wolf's teaching sessions to be planned, assessment data were reviewed.

ASSESSMENT

Basic data about Mr Wolf are contained in Figure 13.1. From initial and subsequent assessments of his ALs, the following data were collected about his normal habits and routines regarding *exercise and rest, weight and diet and sexual activity*.

Data related to exercise/rest:
from assessment of mobilising and sleeping ALs

Usual mobilising habits
Travels to and from work (6 miles return) by car; minimal physical activity during working day; plays golf (2 hours) twice weekly; gardens often very energetically, most weekends

Usual sleeping habits
Goes to bed about 11 pm

Sleeps well midnight–7 am

Does not take sleeping tablets

Never takes a daytime nap

Data related to weight and diet:
from assessment of eating and drinking ALs

Influencing factors
Height 1.8 metres (5 ft 11 in)⎫ ∴ approximately 4.5 kg
Weight 81.6kg (167 lbs)   ⎭ (9 lbs) overweight

Sedentary occupation

No special commendations/restrictions

Finance available for diet modification, if necessary

Habits
Breakfast at 7.30 (cereal, tea, toast with butter and marmalade)

Lunch at 12.30—main meal of the day, with family at weekends and holidays; weekdays at school: soup, meat or fish, vegetables, potatoes/chips, pudding (e.g., custard and tinned fruit)

Supper at 6.30–7.30 (e.g., bacon and egg, bread and biscuits, coffee)

Bedtime snack at 10.30 (milky drink and a biscuit)

Alcohol consumption—minimal during week (e.g., occasional sherry), 2–5 pints beer at weekends, wine with meals occasionally

Dietary likes and dislikes—likes sweet foods, such as puddings

and cakes; takes 2 teaspoonfuls sugar in tea and coffee; enjoys most foods; no particular dislikes

No deliberate restrictions/indulgences

Knowledge
Is aware that diet affects health in various ways; knows he is overweight and feels this may have contributed to his heart disease; considers his drinking habits to be conservative and not dangerous to his health.

Shopping, cooking
Done mainly by wife with his assistance as she requests

Appetite
Always good

Pain, discomforts
None, except occasional mild indigestion following an unusually large meal and occasional discomfort from constipation

Data related to sexual activity
from assessment of the AL of expressing sexuality.

Sexual relationship
Active sexual relationship with wife—sexual intercourse 3 or 4 times a month

No contraception required (wife post-menopause)

No sexual problems/dysfunction

Knowledge/anxieties about effect of current illness on sexual activity
Unsure whether intercourse will now be possible ('Could it bring on a heart attack?')

Thinks his wife will be frightened to resume sexual relations in case this endangers his health

Hopes it will be possible to safely resume normal sexual relations and wishes advice

PLANNING

Having obtained data on which to base the planning of the *content* of the teaching programme, it is now necessary to plan:

- the sequence of teaching sessions
- the timing of the teaching sessions
- the spacing of the teaching sessions
- the method of teaching
- the evaluation of the teaching programme

The sequence of teaching sessions. It may not be very significant in this case but because Mr Wolf is already mobilising and has been worrying about resumption of exercise, it may be most appropriate to begin with the topic of regulation of exercise/rest. As the topic of sexual activity is likely to be the most difficult to discuss with ease and without causing anxiety, it may be best to do that last in the

Patient Assessment Form

Date of admission *8 May*

Date of assessment *8 May*

Surname *WOLF*

Forenames *Henry*

Male [✓]
Female [ ]

Age *54*

Date of birth

Single / *Married* / Widowed [✓]
Other

Prefers to be addressed as

Mr Wolf

Address of usual residence *Cedar Cottage
Anock Village
near Newtown*

Type of accommodation *Country house with ½ acre ground*

Family/Others at this residence *Wife and daughter (age 15)*

Next of kin Name *Mrs Angela Wolf*   Address *as above*

Relationship *Wife*   Tel. no. *Anock 440*

Significant others

Relatives/Dependents *wife and daughter
son (age 20) away at university*

Helpers

Visitors

Occupation *Schoolteacher (languages: county secondary school)*

Religious beliefs and relevant practices *Church of Scotland*

Patient's perception of current health status *Understands he has had a heart attack*

Reason for admission/referral *Myocardial infarction*

Medical diagnosis *Acute anterior M.I.*

Past medical history *Nil of note. No previous hospital admission*

Allergies *None*

Significant life crises
None recent

Fig. 13.1 Mr Wolf: biographical and health data

teaching programme. It is probably useful to include one final session during which previously discussed topics can be revised, further questions raised and points clarified. This allows for the fact that ability to retain information is impaired by anxiety and, therefore, it is to be expected that Mr Wolf will not absorb all of the information first time round. Such a revision session also provides an opportunity for back-up material in written form, such as a booklet or typed sheet, to be given to the patient prior to discharge. Therefore the sequence planned is:

Session	Topic
1	Regulation of exercise/rest
2	Weight and diet
3	Sexual activity
4	Revision/discussion

The timing and spacing of teaching sessions. It is often the practice, when planned teaching is indeed carried out, to present all the information at one time, often immediately prior to discharge. For reasons mentioned above this is not desirable, hence the plan here to provide a series of sessions. With about a week left until discharge, it is feasible to space the 4 sessions planned over several days. In addition, because his wife is to be involved, sessions must be timed to suit her too. Timing each session towards the end of a visiting hour was found to suit Mr and Mrs Wolf and the staff.

The method of teaching. There are many different teaching methods: the formal lecture, audio-visual presentations, the written word in various forms, roleplay, small group discussion. In the case of Mr Wolf, face-to-face discussion is the most appropriate and practicable method. This allows factual information to be given verbally and questions to be asked and answered immediately. The nurse must have considerable skills of establishing rapport and communicating effectively for this method to be successful. She must have her teaching material carefully prepared but, at the same time, be alert to signs from the patient which may indicate the need to repeat something, or develop a topic further, or, if necessary, terminate the session earlier than planned. It may be useful to encourage the patient to make a note of important facts or, alternatively, to provide a summary in writing for him to retain. In Mr Wolf's case, the fact that he is a teacher is an important consideration.

Evaluation of the teaching programme. If any intervention is to be evaluated, goals have to be set at the planning stage of the nursing process. Taking as an example, the third session planned for Mr Wolf on the topic of sexual activity, the goals could be stated as follows:

- ability to assess when it is safe for sexual relations to be resumed

- knowledge of precautions to take before and after intercourse to minimise strain on Mr Wolf's heart
- removal of anxiety and uncertainty about the effect of Mr Wolf's myocardial infarction on sexual relationship

Evaluation of the first 2 goals can be made on the basis of questioning Mr and Mrs Wolf on the details involved at the revision sessions. Evaluation of the third goal may be based on the subjective statements of Mr and Mrs Wolf and an objective observation of their behaviour, in particular the degree of ease with which they become able to talk about the topic of sexual activity.

IMPLEMENTATION

Session 1 Regulation of exercise and rest
Knowing that Mr Wolf already has been feeling that the restrictions imposed on his activity seem to be slowing his progress, it is essential to explain to him the importance of carefully regulating activity and rest. The damaged heart muscle (the myocardium) needs time to heal and this can only take place if demands on the heart are limited and increased very gradually over time. Two to three weeks of minimal activity and maximum rest is necessary, hence the restrictions during the period of hospitalisation. As it takes at least 8 weeks for healing to be completed, physical activity must be limited for that length of time. However, after discharge, it will be important for Mr Wolf to resume activity gradually. Many activities of living, such as personal cleansing and dressing and eating and drinking, are not particularly demanding of energy and so, as long as care is taken to avoid prolonged activity, Mr Wolf will be able to help himself to a considerable degree once at home. Gradually increasing walking is an excellent way of resuming activity e.g., 4 weeks after the myocardial infarction, it should be possible to go out for walks, perhaps about $\frac{1}{4}$ mile every day to begin with; by 10 weeks, a mile (about 20 minutes walking) a day.

As golf is a fairly strenuous form of activity, Mr Wolf should not resume playing until he is able to cope with walking considerable distances. When he does restart he can be advised to begin by playing several holes only, by using a golf caddy in preference to carrying his clubs which is more physically tiring, and by avoiding the stresses of competition golf.

Patients who drive a car are usually advised to refrain from this activity for 3 months or so. As Mrs Wolf also drives, this is not likely to cause too much difficulty, but when Mr Wolf does restart, he should avoid stressful driving.

In the long-term, Mr Wolf's gardening habits are those most likely to require permanent modification. Until his illness, he looked after his $\frac{1}{2}$ acre of ground without assistance and this involved a considerable amount of physical exertion, particularly throughout the summer months. Various suggestions could be put to him:

- to obtain regular help from other members of the family, neighbours or a gardener
- to let part of the ground
- to use power tools where possible
- to make the garden as labour-saving as possible

Fortunately Mr Wolf's job, as a language teacher in a county secondary school, is not excessively demanding of energy and so he is likely to be able to resume work, at least part-time, within 3 months or so. Return to work after a myocardial infarction is considered to be a very important goal, and delaying return too long may cause psychological problems.

In relation to all aspects of regulation of exercise and rest, the important points to communicate are:

- activity must be curtailed to a minimum for 2–3 weeks following a myocardial infarction
- after that time there should be gradual resumption of activity, deliberately planned
- during that period, any sudden or excessive activity must be avoided, so should lifting heavy or cumbersome objects
- walking, gradually increased, is a good form of exercise
- car driving should be avoided for 3 months
- very strenuous activities (e.g., sport or heavy manual work) may need to be avoided permanently
- at any sign of undue exertion (chest pain, breathlessness, dizziness, rapid pulse, palpitations) rest should be taken immediately and that activity avoided.

Session 2 Weight and diet

The goal for a person who has suffered a myocardial infarction should be to keep his weight near, and preferably a little below, the average for his height and build. Mr Wolf is approximately 4.5 kg (9 lbs) overweight, so a weight-reducing diet aimed at a loss of 6 kg (approximately 12 lbs) might be a realistic target in the short-term, perhaps a period of 2–3 months.

Reviewing Mr Wolf's normal eating and drinking habits (p. 102) indicates a number of possible targets for weight-reduction: reducing or avoiding sugar in hot drinks; avoiding bread (except minimum amount of wholemeal bread) and biscuits; cutting down on weekend beer intake; and replacing weekday puddings with a piece of fresh fruit. Probably doing all or most of these would be sufficient to achieve the relatively small weight loss required.

It is likely that Mrs Wolf will be enthusiastic about assisting her husband in this way and, if she requests it, a more detailed diet sheet might be obtained from the hospital dietitian.

Because of the association between coronary artery disease and heart attacks, people who have suffered a myocardial infarction are generally advised to take unsaturated rather than saturated fats in order to reduce the amount of cholesterol in the diet.[1] This can be achieved by the following dietary modifications: eating less meat, removing fat from meat, grilling rather than frying meat; using a soft margarine high in polyunsaturated fat for spreading and cooking instead of butter or other margarine; using oils high in polyunsaturated fat; avoiding cream, keeping cheese intake low, eating a maximum of 3 eggs per week.

It will be reassuring to both Mr and Mrs Wolf that it is reduction in fat and kilojoule intake over time that matters, rather than at every single meal. Special meals can still be enjoyed on occasions.

Session 3 Sexual activity

It is clear that Mr Wolf has anxieties about this topic, and that he suspects his wife will have too. First and foremost the nurse should convey to the couple that these anxieties are very common and that, just like exercise and diet, there are clear guidelines which can be provided to answer the uncertainties they may have.

As most people are aware, sexual intercourse makes considerable demands on the heart. The pulse rate may rise from 70 to as high as 180 beats per minute, the blood pressure from 120 to over 250, and the respiratory rate from 16 to more than 40 per minute. However, there is general agreement among cardiologists that sexual activity is compatible with heart disease as long as the patient knows how to assess his ability and learn to identify warning signs of heart strain. Puksta (1977) provides excellent guidelines about the kind of advice which nurses could give to a post-coronary patient. It may be safe for sexual relations to be resumed within a few weeks (perhaps as soon as 4 weeks after discharge i.e., almost 2 months after the MI occurred). Readiness to do so can be assessed on the patient's ability to perform exercises of comparable physical exertion. A useful guide is what is referred to as the 'stair-climbing test': the energy cost for sexual intercourse is equal to climbing two flights of stairs at a brisk rate (within a minute). Mr Wolf can be reassured that it is very unusual for intercourse to result in a fatal heart attack. It is also possible for the patient to learn to recognise the warning signs of heart strain from sexual intercourse, and thus reduce exertion. These signs include: rapid pulse and respiration rate persisting 30 minutes after intercourse; palpitations 15 minutes after; chest pain during or after; exhaustion following intercourse or extreme fatigue the next day.

Advice can also be given on when to avoid sexual intercourse: soon after a large meal or alcohol consumption; in an extremely hot or cold environment; in an anxiety-provoking situation; and if other strenuous activity is planned to follow.

[1] Increasingly there is controversy over this point. For further discussion see Thompson, 1980.

Finally Mr and Mrs Wolf can be reassured that sexual activity between long-married couples is, in fact, less strenuous than many other activities, such as driving a car or having an argument!

EVALUATION

As mentioned in the discussion of the planning phase of the teaching programme (p. 104), goals have to be set in order for evaluation to be possible. There follows, in summary form, the goals that could be stated as the outcome of the 3 teaching sessions:

Session   Goals

1.   Exercise and rest

Understanding need for limitation on physical exercise (maximum rest in the initial recovery period)

Understanding need for gradual resumption of physical exercise

Formulation of plan of exercise resumption

Confirmation that Mr and Mrs Wolf no longer feel anxious or uncertain about exercise/rest requirements

2.   Weight and diet

Agreement on need for Mr Wolf to reduce weight by approximately 6 kg

Understanding how to achieve that weight loss in a 2–3 month period

Expressing motivation to do above

Understanding reason for reducing cholesterol intake and knowing how to achieve it

3.   Sexual activity

Understanding how to assess when it is safe for sexual relations to be resumed

Knowing what precautions to take before and after intercourse to minimise strain on Mr Wolf's heart

Removing anxiety and uncertainty about the effect of Mr Wolf's MI on their sexual relationship

The teaching programme described for Mr Wolf is, of course, only part of the teaching component of his rehabilitation. In the period immediately following his admission to the Coronary Care Unit, teaching was going on, albeit unplanned, as the doctors and nurses answered Mr Wolf's various questions. Then, following his discharge, further teaching by the general practitioner or community nurse will be necessary as the patient and his wife realise they need other information and support, or as unanticipated difficulties arise.

It is not common practice for nurses to carry out patient teaching in the planned way described in this chapter, but the advantages of so doing should be obvious.

Why do nurses *not* participate in patients' rehabilitation in this way? It may be because nurses have been slow to appreciate how important is the teaching component of their job or perhaps they feel it is the doctor's responsibility rather than theirs. It is, as mentioned earlier a shared responsibility.

Many readers, although convinced that patients should be taught as Mr Wolf was, will say that it is not possible because it is too time-consuming. Of course, it does take time to plan and implement a teaching programme. However, it is time well-spent and, after the initial work a generalised plan formulated could readily be modified to suit individual patients.

REFERENCES

Puksta N S 1979 All about sex . . . after a coronary. American Journal of Nursing 77 (4) April: 602–605

Thompson D R 1980 Fats and heart disease: a point for controversy. Nursing Times 76 (31) July: 1360–1361

Postscript

Although throughout the text each presentation dealt with a particular aspect of the process of nursing, it cannot be too strongly stressed that in the nursing of any one patient, *all* aspects of the process must be thought through and applied.

Furthermore each presentation dealt with a circumscribed time period related to the patient's individual circumstances in order to illustrate application of the selected aspect of the process of nursing. But in reality there has to be updating of a patient's nursing records during the *continuous period of time* in which he requires nursing.

On the next few pages there are seveal blank Patient Assessment Forms to help readers to develop a way of using the process, based on the Roper, Logan and Tierney model for nursing illustrated in this book. It is hoped that readers will practise collecting information in a similar way, starting with a patient's biographical and health data, then relevant information about his everyday living, particularly what he can and cannot do in relation to his ALs; and from these data to compile a list of his health problems, both actual and potential.

Learners can then proceed to practise documenting the other phases of the process—planning, implementation and evaluation—on whatever stationery is provided for the patients' nursing records. Practising the process mode of thinking about nursing does not require special stationery.

Patient Assessment Form

Date of admission   Date of assessment

Surname   Forenames

Male ☐   Age ☐   Single/Married/Widowed   Prefers to be addressed as
Female ☐   Other

                          Date of birth

Address of usual residence

Type of accommodation

Family/Others at this residence

Next of kin   Name   Address

                     Relationship   Tel. no.

Significant others   Relatives/Dependents

                          Helpers

                          Visitors

Occupation

Religious beliefs and relevant practices

Patient's perception of current health status

Reason for admission/referral

Medical diagnosis

Past medical history

Allergies   Significant life crises

Assessment of Activities of Living

Date

AL	Usual routines: what he/she can and cannot do independently	Patient's problems (actual/potential) (p) = potential
● Maintaining a safe environment		
● Communicating		
● Breathing		
● Eating and drinking		
● Eliminating		
● Personal cleansing and dressing		
● Controlling body temperature		
● Mobilising		
● Working and playing		
● Expressing sexuality		
● Sleeping		
● Dying		

Patient Assessment Form

Date of admission

Date of assessment

Surname

Forenames

Male ☐

Female ☐

Age ☐

Date of birth

Single/Married/Widowed

Other

Prefers to be addressed as

Address of usual residence

Type of accommodation

Family/Others at this residence

Next of kin

Name

Address

Relationship

Tel. no.

Significant others

Relatives/Dependents

Helpers

Visitors

Occupation

Religious beliefs and relevant practices

Patient's perception of current health status

Reason for admission/referral

Medical diagnosis

Past medical history

Allergies

Significant life crises

Assessment of Activities of Living

Date

Patient's problems
(actual/potential)
(p) = potential

AL

Usual routines:
what he/she can and cannot do independently

● Maintaining
a safe
environment

● Communicating

● Breathing

● Eating and
drinking

● Eliminating

● Personal
cleansing and
dressing

● Controlling
body
temperature

● Mobilising

● Working
and playing

● Expressing
sexuality

● Sleeping

● Dying

Patient Assessment Form

Date of admission

Date of assessment

Surname

Forenames

Male ☐

Female ☐

Age ☐

Date of birth

Single/Married/Widowed

Other

Prefers to be addressed as

Address of usual residence

Type of accommodation

Family/Others at this residence

Next of kin

Name

Relationship

Address

Tel. no.

Significant others

Relatives/Dependents

Helpers

Visitors

Occupation

Religious beliefs and relevant practices

Patient's perception of current health status

Reason for admission/referral

Medical diagnosis

Past medical history

Allergies

Significant life crises

Assessment of Activities of Living

Date

AL

Usual routines:
what he/she can and cannot do independently

Patient's problems
(actual/potential)
(p) = potential

- Maintaining
  a safe
  environment

- Communicating

- Breathing

- Eating and
  drinking

- Eliminating

- Personal
  cleansing and
  dressing

- Controlling
  body
  temperature

- Mobilising

- Working
  and playing

- Expressing
  sexuality

- Sleeping

- Dying

Patient Assessment Form

Date of admission

Date of assessment

Surname

Forenames

Male ☐

Age ☐

Single/Married/Widowed

Prefers to be addressed as

Female ☐

Other

Date of birth

Address of usual residence

Type of accommodation

Family/Others at this residence

Next of kin | Name | Address

Relationship | Tel. no.

Significant others | Relatives/Dependents

Helpers

Visitors

Occupation

Religious beliefs and relevant practices

Patient's perception of current health status

Reason for admission/referral

Medical diagnosis

Past medical history

Allergies | Significant life crises

Assessment of Activities of Living

Date

Patient's problems
(actual/potential)
(p) = potential

AL

Usual routines:
what he/she can and cannot do independently

● Maintaining
a safe
environment

● Communicating

● Breathing

● Eating and
drinking

● Eliminating

● Personal
cleansing and
dressing

● Controlling
body
temperature

● Mobilising

● Working
and playing

● Expressing
sexuality

● Sleeping

● Dying

Patient Assessment Form

Date of admission   Date of assessment

Surname   Forenames

Male ☐   Age ☐   Single/Married/Widowed   Prefers to be addressed as

Female ☐   Other

Date of birth

Address of usual residence

Type of accommodation

Family/Others at this residence

Next of kin   Name   Address

                     Relationship   Tel. no.

Significant others   Relatives/Dependents

                     Helpers

                     Visitors

Occupation

Religious beliefs and relevant practices

Patient's perception of current health status

Reason for admission/referral

Medical diagnosis

Past medical history

Allergies   Significant life crises

Assessment of Activities of Living

Date

Patient's problems
(actual/potential)
(p) = potential

AL | Usual routines:
what he/she can and cannot do independently

● Maintaining
a safe
environment

● Communicating

● Breathing

● Eating and
drinking

● Eliminating

● Personal
cleansing and
dressing

● Controlling
body
temperature

● Mobilising

● Working
and playing

● Expressing
sexuality

● Sleeping

● Dying

Patient Assessment Form

Date of admission   Date of assessment

Surname   Forenames

Male ☐   Age ☐   Single/Married/Widowed   Prefers to be addressed as
Female ☐   Other

                          Date of birth

Address of usual residence

Type of accommodation

Family/Others at this residence

Next of kin   Name   Address

                     Relationship   Tel. no.

Significant others   Relatives/Dependents

                          Helpers

                          Visitors

Occupation

Religious beliefs and relevant practices

Patient's perception of current health status

Reason for admission/referral

Medical diagnosis

Past medical history

Allergies   Significant life crises

Assessment of Activities of Living

Date

AL	Usual routines: what he/she can and cannot do independently	Patient's problems (actual/potential) (p) = potential

● Maintaining
a safe
environment

● Communicating

● Breathing

● Eating and
drinking

● Eliminating

● Personal
cleansing and
dressing

● Controlling
body
temperature

● Mobilising

● Working
and playing

● Expressing
sexuality

● Sleeping

● Dying